# Nursing Diagnoses for Wellness
## Supporting Strengths

**Arlene DeGangi Houldin,** R.N., M.S.N.
    Associate Professor
    Thomas Jefferson University
    College of Allied Health Sciences
    Department of Nursing
    Philadelphia, PA


**Susan Walls Saltstein,** R.N., M.S.N., C.P.N.P.
    Assistant Professor
    Thomas Jefferson University
    College of Allied Health Sciences
    Department of Nursing
    Philadelphia, PA


**Kathleen Marie Ganley,** R.N., M.S.N.
    Assistant Professor
    Thomas Jefferson University
    College of Allied Health Sciences
    Department of Nursing
    Philadelphia, PA

# Nursing Diagnoses
## for Wellness
### Supporting Strengths

**J. B. Lippincott Company    Philadelphia**

London    Mexico City    New York
St. Louis    São Paulo    Sydney

Sponsoring Editor: Diana Intenzo
Manuscript Editor: Marjory I. Fraser
Indexer: Angela Holt
Art Director: Tracy Baldwin
Design Coordinator: Anne O'Donnell
Designer: Susan Hess
Production Manager: Kathleen P. Dunn
Production Coordinator: Les Hoeltzel
Compositor: University Graphics
Printer/Binder: RR Donnelley & Sons Company

6   5

**Library of Congress Cataloging-in-Publication Data**

Houldin, Arlene DeGangi.
    Nursing diagnoses for wellness.
    Includes bibliographies and index.
    1. Diagnosis—Handbooks, manuals, etc.   2. Nursing—
Handbooks, manuals, etc.   3. Health status indicators—
Handbooks, manuals, etc.   4. Nursing care plans—Handbooks,
manuals, etc.   I. Saltstein, Susan Walls.   II. Ganley, Kathleen
Marie.   III. Title.   [DNLM: 1. Health Promotion—nurses'
instruction.   2. Nursing Process.   3. Patient Care Planning. WY
100 H8383n]
RT48.H68, 1987        610.73        86-20067
ISBN 0-397-54645-9

# Preface

Health promotion and illness/accident prevention are integral parts of the professional nurse's role in delivering the highest quality of nursing care to the consumer.

*Nursing Diagnoses for Wellness: Supporting Strengths* presents wellness-oriented nursing diagnoses to be utilized in prescribing interventions and/or learning activities for both the well and the ill client in any setting. These wellness-related diagnoses emphasize strengths that should be identified and enhanced to achieve the highest level of wellness possible for the client.

The authors have presented information necessary for systematic identification and analysis of the healthy aspect(s) of client functioning.

These wellness-oriented nursing diagnoses are based on an extensive review of literature, clinical observation, and practice. These diagnoses meet a need for recognition and utilization of client strengths that has not been met in the official North American Nursing Diagnoses Association (NANDA) listing. The current nursing diagnoses from the NANDA listing are included in their entirety in the text.

The handbook is organized according to functional health patterns and describes each nursing diagnosis in terms of health status, contributing factors, and defining characteristics. Several care plans are written to apply the wellness-oriented nursing diagnoses in a variety of situations. These wellness-related diagnoses are not meant to be an exhaustive list but should serve rather as a focus for wellness, with additional wellness diagnoses, generated as needed by each individual client situation.

The authors recognize that as these nursing diagnoses are tested and utilized in practice situations, additional information will be generated to refine and expand these wellness-related nursing diagnoses.

Arlene DeGangi Houldin, R.N., M.S.N.
Susan Walls Saltstein, R.N., M.S.N., C.P.N.P.
Kathleen Marie Ganley, R.N., M.S.N.

# *Acknowledgments*

The authors wish to thank their families and friends for the support and encouragement offered. We want to thank our husbands Thomas McVeigh, Elliott Saltstein, and Frank Houldin for their patience and understanding. In particular, gratitude is extended to Frank Houldin for his editing and critique of the manuscript. Thank you to Lillian and Anthony DeGangi. Their assistance helped make this book a successful endeavor.

Special thanks to our children Kate, Scott, Mark, and Ryan, who make everything possible.

We extend our gratitude to Lynda Carpenito for her support and critical review of the manuscript. Our appreciation is offered to Diana Intenzo, Editor-in-Chief, Nursing Division, JB Lippincott Company, for her guidance and understanding.

We are grateful to Renée McCain for her excellent typing skills and diligent efforts.

# Contents

## Section II: Wellness-Oriented Nursing Diagnoses Grouped by Functional Health Patterns

### *Functional Pattern 1: Health Perception— Health Management*

### *Functional Pattern 2: Nutrition—Metabolic*

## Section III: Case Studies/Care Plans

# I
# Overview

# Introduction

The problem-solving methodology utilized by nurses to deliver professional services includes the acquisition of data concerning the health status of an individual, family, or community. Analysis of these facts results in a specific statement that identifies an existing or potential health problem. This statement is referred to as the nursing diagnosis and provides the focus for the nurse's plan of care. Currently accepted nursing diagnosis categories are centered around the actual or potentially deleterious effects of illness on the health status of clients. The classification, publication, and use of these illness-oriented nursing diagnosis categories has greatly enhanced the credibility and autonomy ascribed to professional nursing practice in recent years.

Decision-making and therapeutic intervention strategies initiated by nurses are not, however, limited to the treatment of problems identified in the most recent nursing diagnoses approved at the Seventh National Conference on Classification of Nursing Diagnosis (see the box, Approved Nursing Diagnoses [North American Nursing Diagnosis Association, April, 1986]). Rather, professional nursing practice focuses on assisting individuals and groups to attain their optimal health potential and to meet their health care needs. Although there has been a long history of professed nursing commitment to the promotion of health and the prevention of illness, the emphasis of nursing education and practice, in many instances, has been on recognition and intervention in illness.

As nurse educators, interested in teaching nursing students to promote health, prevent illness, and capitalize on clients' strengths, we have repeatedly la-

*Text continues on page 9*

## *APPROVED NURSING DIAGNOSES (NORTH AMERICAN NURSING DIAGNOSIS ASSOCIATION, APRIL 1986)*

Activity intolerance
Activity intolerance, potential
Adjustment, impaired*
Airway clearance, ineffective
Anxiety
Body temperature, potential alteration in*
Bowel elimination, alteration in: constipation
Bowel elimination, alteration in: diarrhea
Bowel elimination, alteration in: incontinence
Breathing pattern, ineffective
Cardiac output, alteration in: decreased
Comfort, alteration in: pain
Comfort, alteration in: chronic pain*
Communication, impaired: verbal
Coping, family: potential for growth
Coping, ineffective family: compromised

continued

Coping, ineffective family: disabling
Coping, ineffective individual
Diversional activity, deficit
Family process, alteration in
Fear
Fluid volume alteration in: excess
Fluid volume deficit, actual
Fluid volume deficit, potential
Gas exchange, impaired
Grieving, anticipatory
Grieving, dysfunctional
Growth and development, altered*
Health maintenance, alteration in
Home maintenance management, impaired
Hopelessness*
Hyperthermia*
Hypothermia*
Incontinence, functional*
Incontinence, reflex*
Incontinence, stress*
Incontinence, total*
Infection, potential for*

Injury, potential for: (poisoning, potential for; suf-
     focation, potential for; trauma, potential for)
Knowledge deficit (specify)
Mobility, impaired physical
Noncompliance (specify)
Nutrition, alteration in: less than body
     requirements
Nutrition, alteration in: more than body
     requirements
Nutrition, alteration in: potential for more than
     body requirements
Oral mucous membrane, alteration in
Parenting, alteration in: actual
Parenting, alteration in: potential
Post trauma response*
Powerlessness
Rape trauma syndrome
Self-care deficit: feeding, bathing/hygiene, dress-
     ing/grooming, toileting
Self-concept, disturbance in body image, self-es-
     teem, role performance, personal identity

continued

Sensory-perceptual alteration: visual, auditory,
     kinesthetic, gustatory, tactile, olfactory
Sexual dysfunction
Sexuality patterns, altered*
Skin integrity, impairment of: actual
Skin integrity, impairment of: potential
Sleep pattern disturbance
Social interaction, impaired*
Social isolation
Spiritual distress (distress of the human spirit)
Swallowing, impaired*
Thermoregulation, ineffective*
Thought processes, alteration in
Tissue integrity, impaired*
Tissue perfusion, alteration in: cerbral, cardio-
     pulmonary, renal, gastrointestinal,
     peripheral
Unilateral neglect
Urinary elimination, alteration in patterns
Urinary retention*
Violence, potential for: self-directed or directed

*Diagnoses accepted in 1986.

(Etiology and Defining Characteristics of Nursing Diagnoses can be found in: Gebbie K, Lavin MA (ed): Summary of the First National Conference. St. Louis, CV Mosby, 1973; Gebbie K (ed): Summary of the Second National Conference. Clearinghouse for Nursing Diagnosis (out of print); Kim MJ, Moritz D (eds): Classification of Nursing Diagnoses: Proceedings of the Third and Fourth National Conferences. New York, McGraw–Hill, 1982; Kim MJ, McFarland GK, McLane AM (eds): Classification of Nursing Diagnoses: Proceedings of the Fifth National Conference. St. Louis, CV Mosby, 1984; Hurley M (ed): Classification of Nursing Diagnoses: Proceedings of the Sixth Conference. St. Louis, CV Mosby, 1986; McLane AM (ed): Classification of Nursing Diagnoses: Proceedings of the Seventh Conference. St. Louis, CV Mosby (in press)

mented the fact that no identification or classification of wellness-related diagnoses is available in the literature. Our nursing students are forced to rely on a haphazard, nonspecific classification method to identify and incorporate client strengths into their nursing care planning.

Whether the nursing goal is to maintain and promote health activities, prevent illness, identify acute or chronic needs/problems, or support the client in meeting death with dignity, identification and analysis of the strengths of the client is imperative to provide comprehensive, meaningful nursing care. Almost every client, no matter how critically or chronically ill, has strengths. This healthy aspect of client functioning must be recognized, identified, and mobilized to assist the client in reaching the highest possible level of functioning or in meeting death with dignity.

The purpose of this book is to begin to systematically identify health/wellness behaviors and to demonstrate how nursing interventions can be written to maintain and capitalize on identified client strengths, for every client in every setting. There is a tremendous need for continuing research, refinement, and dissemination of information in this critical area of health-enhancement activities. We cannot wait, however, for optimum solutions before beginning to act to fill a void that exists in the provision of comprehensive care to clients.

At this point, the definition of commonly used terms will be discussed. The term *client* will be used in this book because of its application to individuals and groups who are essentially well.

Various definitions of nursing diagnosis have evolved in the past 25 to 30 years. For the purpose of this text the definition of nursing diagnosis is based on Bircher's definition (1975). "A nursing diagnosis is a statement of a client's unique health status which is derived from nursing assessment based on all factors affecting his well-being, dignity, rights, recovery, maintenance, promotion of health and attainment of a meaningful life-style." Therefore, a nursing diagnosis considers five realms of experience and knowledge: the biological, physical-environmental, sociocultural, psychological, and spiritual realms.

The term *health promotion* refers to activities directed toward developing the resources of clients that maintain or enhance well-being. The term *prevention* refers to activities that seek to protect clients from potential or actual health threats and their harmful consequences.

# Changing Trends in Health Care

## Health Maintenance

Historically, the focus of health care has been on the curing of disease and the treatment of illness in traditional settings such as the hospital. Presently, there is a growing emphasis on health promotion, disease prevention, and optimal functioning for all persons, including the chronically ill and disabled. Early hospital discharge and reliance on home care by family members and community-based support services clearly reflect the need for comprehensive health care services. Preventative health care that includes screening and health promotion and protection programs are expected services now being sought by the consumer. In order to meet these changing health care demands, the nurse must be cognizant of the total health and available strengths of clients that support sound health care practices, recovery from illness, and optimal physical and psychological functioning.

The current health care reimbursement pattern accentuates the rapid movement of clients through the health care system. The need for mobilizing client resources in meeting health care needs in hospital, ambulatory, and home care settings is evident. Obviously, the strengths of the client must be systematically identified and utilized to promote client independence. Nurses must assume responsibility for assisting clients to achieve competence in self-care activities whenever possible. We are at the cutting edge of an evolution of health care practices. Nurses must assume leadership in providing the tools and interventions relevant to clients' changing health care needs.

Health planning priorities of governmental, private sector, and consumer agencies now include the development of programs for community health education. Health counseling, anticipatory guidance, stress management, health-risk appraisal, and lifestyle modification are now considered essential for comprehensive health care delivery. The growth of the concept of maintaining wellness, as opposed to treating illness, is clearly evident in the successful operation of thousands of health maintenance organizations (HMO) throughout the country. Elimination of health-risk behaviors and life-style modification for the purpose of improving health status are currently being rewarded in the workplace. Incentives are being offered to employees who choose to utilize information for improving their health status. It is well known that exercise, proper nutrition, and effective management of stress can significantly reduce morbidity and mortality in all age groups. Health promotion and illness prevention efforts not only enhance the longevity and quality of life, but also reduce health care costs and increase productivity associated with reduced illness and absenteeism.

Nursing is charged with the responsibility for rendering comprehensive health care services that include health promotion and illness prevention activities. These activities are carried out on a continuing basis in all health care settings. Nurses have become increasingly more visible and vital to the collaborative planning and implementation of health care services by virtue of their education, experience, and expertise. Nursing assessment and analysis activities must be directed toward identification of the often unrecognized potential in individuals and families for assuming self-care for better personal health. Documentation of these potentials can significantly influence health care policies and trends that support healthy life-styles. Nursing diagnosis statements that define motivational and wellness behaviors, as identified in this handbook, must be integrated into the nursing professional's present approach to care planning in order to achieve the goals of health promotion and prevention of illness.

## Holistic Approach to Health Care

The recognition of the individual as a whole person, that is, one who possesses the physical, psychological, and social potential for optimal functioning throughout life, is central to the practice of professional nursing. Health promotion activities focus on the development of these potentials as resources that restore, maintain, or enhance well-being. Nurses recognize that illness is not inevitable and that an orientation toward the future acquisition of physiologic and psychosocial need satisfaction is the ultimate goal of holistic nursing practice. This holistic approach to health care by nurses includes the recognition of professional responsibility to facilitate and support the health-seeking behaviors and basic potential for fulfillment in all individuals.

The presence of illness or disease can significantly alter an individual's ability to maintain functional health. Problem identification in the form of nursing diagnosis provides the focus for nursing interventions that address need satisfaction. Illness and problem identification should not, however, be the primary focus for care planning. This would be inconsistent with holistic nursing practice and detrimental to the health promotional goals of comprehensive care. Nurses, although responsible for problem solving, need also to place an equal emphasis on promoting health.

It is imperative that nurses utilize a classification of wellness-related diagnoses, as well as illness-related diagnoses, to accurately identify the needs of each client. The recognition and assessment of the unique configuration of the needs and strengths of clients allows the nurse to mobilize the health aspect of the client in addition to identifying needs and problems that require nursing intervention.

---

## Orientation Toward Wellness in Nursing Diagnosis

The use of wellness-oriented nursing diagnosis serves several purposes. Both the nurse and the consumer of nursing services are encouraged to examine those positive, adaptive, or previously successful behaviors that contribute to identified healthy functioning. These behaviors, written as nursing diagnosis statements of wellness, can then be utilized to reinforce continued health promotion and protection as well as avenues for addressing problem-solving in the case of illness, adaptation to disability or toward a dignified death.

The incorporation of health-related nursing diagnosis statements into care planning can also be viewed as an opportunity for nursing professionals to expand their contribution to long-term health outcomes. Assessment of strengths and health-promoting behaviors, shared and supported in collaboration with the recipient of nursing care, encourages the continued use of positive strategies in similar circumstances.

Wellness-oriented nursing diagnosis, by facilitating positive outcomes for the consumer of health care, serves to promote the best possible professional health care delivery. Nurses in primary care settings (clinic, doctors' offices, health maintenance organizations, schools, community health facilities, geriatric centers, and industrial health programs) can use these diagnoses to identify and maintain sound health practices and resources for health promotion and protection because problem-oriented diagnoses are often inappropriate when caring for a basically healthy population. Nurses who provide services in secondary care settings (nursing homes, rehabilitation centers, community hospitals, and mental health residential homes) can incorporate wellness-oriented diagnosis to redirect planning for early discharge and strengthen home management. Tertiary care nurses can utilize positive statements of analysis to support recovery and family participation in care delivery.

Essentially, this handbook describes factors that contribute to positive health status and conditions. The nursing diagnosis statements listed in the box, "Nursing Diagnosis List Grouped Under Functional Health Patterns," are grouped according to the functional health patterns identified by M. Gordon (*Nursing Diagnosis: Process and Application*. New York, McGraw–Hill, 1982) and L. Carpenito (*Handbook of Nursing Diagnosis*. Philadelphia, JB

## NURSING DIAGNOSIS LIST GROUPED UNDER FUNCTIONAL HEALTH PATTERNS

| *Functional Pattern* | *Diagnosis* |
| --- | --- |
| 1. Health perception Health management | Health maintenance, appropriate<br>Accident prevention practices, adequate |
| 2. Nutritional— Metabolic | Nutritional status, optimal<br>Fluid volume, adequate<br>Immune response, effective<br>Skin integrity, adequate |
| 3. Elimination | Bowel elimination, adequate<br>Bladder elimination, adequate |

| | |
|---|---|
| 4. Activity exercise | Activity tolerance |
| | Physical fitness, optimal |
| | Respiratory function, effective |
| | Cardiac functioning, effective |
| | Home maintenance management, effective |
| | Self-care, independence |
| 5. Sleep—Rest | Sleep pattern, adequate |
| 6. Cognitive— Perceptual | Developmental progression, efficient |
| | Potential for successful satisfaction of developmental needs |
| | Comfort, adequate |

continued

| 7. Self-perception | Stress response, adaptive |
| | Self-concept, positive |
| | Body image, positive |
| | Self-esteem, adequate |
| 8. Role— Relationship | Coping, effective family |
| | Social interaction, satisfactory |
| 9. Sexuality— Reproductive | Sexual function, adequate |
| 10. Coping—Stress Tolerance | Crisis resolution, effective |
| | Coping, effective individual |
| 11. Value—Belief | Spiritual support |

(Adapted from Carpenito LJ: *Handbook of Nursing Diagnosis*. Philadelphia, JB Lippincott, 1984)

Lippincott, 1984) with some minor changes. The nursing diagnosis statements include a brief definition of the health need as it has been satisifed when applicable. The statement is then divided into two parts as has been described by numerous other authors. Part I (Health Status) of the statement describes the actual or potential wellnesss state of the individual or family. Part II (Contributing Factors) of the statement consists of a list of healthy behaviors or sound health practices that influence or contribute to the particular healthy or well aspect of the client's status or functioning. The third aspect of the nursing diagnosis (defining characteristics) includes a list of possible or probable findings that provide evidence to support the nursing diagnosis.

Prior to identifying the nursing diagnosis that best describes the client's health status, the nurse gathers a comprehensive data base of assessment information that addresses a particular functional health pattern category. This assessment phase, vital to nursing process methodology, should be carefully followed when determining a wellness-oriented nursing diagnosis. This procedure ensures accurate analysis and appropriate assignment of a nursing diagnosis to the individual or family who possesses the potential or exhibits an area(s) of strength or sound health practice in a particular functional health pattern. Included in the appendix in this handbook is an assessment tool designed to elicit information about the health promotional or protective functioning of an individual or family. The nurse who uses this tool is encouraged to utilize previous knowledge and experience in assessment modalities to secure comprehensive and accurate data.

Preparation and investigation of the wellness-oriented nursing diagnosis statements listed in this handbook revealed several etiological or contributing factors that are applicable to several different functional health pattern categories. These factors are recognized as strengths that may be present at some level in all persons or groups. A list of those contributing factors considered to be relevant to all aspects of health functioning is found in the box, Commonly Identified Factors That Contribute to Wellness. They can be incorporated into a specific nursing diagnosis statement as contributing factors. The nurse may choose to add these statements as adjunct factors to ensure individuality and specificity in the assignment of a nursing diagnosis.

## COMMONLY IDENTIFIED FACTORS THAT CONTRIBUTE TO WELLNESS

Realistic self-concept
Acceptance of self
Accurate perception of reality
Autonomous functioning
Strong ethical sense
Responsibility for own actions
Self-direction
Adaptability
Creativity
Ability to express feelings
Effective problem-solving ability
Capacity for abstract thought
Sense of industry
Self-respect
Respect for needs of others
Scholastic (work) achievement
Insightful behavior
Role satisfaction
Effective social involvement

Satisfying interpersonal relationships
Ability to cope with illness
Ability to accept need for dependency
Positive role models
Physical capability
Effective management of disabilities
Accurate and sufficient information
Ability to accept the independent/dependent
    needs of others
Feelings of competence
Effective management of stressors (divorce, sepa-
    ration, illness, death, and so forth)
Ability to grieve appropriately
Appropriate sense of humor
Adequate support systems
Availabiilty of adequate resources (financial, cog-
    nitive, educational and physical)
Sense of well-being
Political awareness and associated activities re-
    lated to health and safety concerns
Desire to learn
Internal locus of control

# Formulation of Nursing Diagnosis

A correctly written nursing diagnosis provides efficiency, organization, and clarity when communicating with clients, nurses, and other health care providers.

In order to formulate an accurate diagnosis, assessment data must be carefully gathered and analyzed. Nurses must ensure that the nursing diagnosis is supported by assessment data. Valid information obtained by cues must not be confused with biases or prejudices obtained by inference. Certain accurate inferences, however, can be made based on a solid foundation of information.

A *cue* is defined as a single unit of noticed information received through the senses and described as objectively, accurately, and precisely as possible.

An inference is defined as the nurse's subjective, personal meanings assigned to the situation based on cues or groups of cues (see box, Examples of Cues and Inferences). The nurse must be careful not to use judgments about the situation as though they were the actual situation.

## Purpose of the Nursing Diagnosis

To identify the problem or health status of the client. Nursing diagnosis gives focus and direction to nursing actions.

## Types of Diagnoses

1. *Actual*—the condition presently producing difficulty or the current health status of the client. It is observed by the nurse or stated by the client.

2. *Potential*—condition or altered state that does not presently exist but may develop or become an actual diagnosis. Potential can describe a capacity for growth or for deterioration of health status.

3. *Possible*—the condition with a high probability of developing because of changes of the existing condition or diagnosis (medical). This can also describe conditions that may be present but that require additional data to confirm or rule out.

## Components of the Nursing Diagnosis

The diagnostic statement has two main phrases with a connecting phrase.

1. *The Problem Statement*—describes an alteration or condition that is actual/potential/possible (describes the present state of the existing problem or health status).

Suggestion: check the list of accepted Nursing Diagnoses (see the box, Approved Nursing Diagnoses [North American Diagnosis Association, April 1986] and the diagnoses for wellness listed in this book). Choose the category most appropriate for your client, based on the data gathered and analyzed. Specify for the individual client situation as needed.

a. Descriptive modifiers can be used as needed (*e.g.*, mild/moderate/severe).

b. Keep the descriptive statement as concise as possible.

2. *The Connecting Phrase*— expresses the relationship between the two main phrases. Use of the terms "associated with" and "related to" is recommended. Avoid use of the terms "due to" and "as a result of" because these imply a cause-and-effect relationship that might be difficult to establish with certainty. These

phrases also place the legal burden of proof of this cause-and-effect relationship on the nurse.

3. *The Basis/Reason Phrase*—suggests a cause or reason for the alteration or condition. Make this part of the diagnostic statement as specific and concise as possible.

4. The inclusion of the phrase "as evidenced by" is optional. It can be utilized to enumerate the specific supporting evidence for the diagnosis.

---

## Things to Include in Nursing Diagnosis

1. State the nursing diagnosis in terms of conclusions reached from valid and accurate nursing assessment data.

2. The conclusions should not include a re-statement of the medical diagnosis or pathology or treatments prescribed.

3. Separate unrelated diagnoses even though the supporting data may be similar.

4. Use legally acceptable nonjudgmental language in writing the diagnoses.

5. Do not lump unrelated alterations or conditions together even though the etiology of the alteration may be the same. Goals and interventions are likely to be different for individual alterations.

6. Avoid legally inadvisable or judgmental statements (*e.g.*, fear related to frequent beatings from her husband, or potential alternation in parenting associated with the low IQ of the mother).

## *Differences Between Medical and Nursing Diagnoses*

The differences between medical and nursing diagnoses reflect differing goals. Medical diagnoses focus on pathology, treatment, cure of disease, or reduction of injury. If the disorder cannot be identified, frequently the signs or symptoms of the condition or situation are treated.

Nursing diagnosis focuses on the client's response to illness or other factors that adversely affect, or have the potential to adversely affect, the attainment or maintenance of optimal wellness. Nursing diagnosis can also refer to a client's health status. It is not necessary to have a medical diagnosis before a nursing diagnosis can be formulated.

| MEDICAL DIAGNOSIS | NURSING DIAGNOSIS* |
| --- | --- |
| Diabetes | Impaired skin integrity (ulcer of the dorsal aspect of the first right toe) related to vascular changes of diabetes |
| | Knowledge deficit related to dietary requirements in diabetes |
| Fractured right femur | Alteration in comfort (pain) associated with a fracture of the right femur |
| | Impaired physical mobility related to a fracture of the right femur |

*Adapted from Yoder ME: Introduction to Nursing Diagnosis. Philadelphia, JB Lippincott, 1985.

A nursing diagnosis is made in collaboration with the client. The diagnoses continually evolve and necessitate reassessment and change during the nurse–client contact.

The first step in the formulation of a nursing diagnosis is the identification of the client's health status, concerns, or needs. If the client is well, with or without a medical diagnosis, and is coping adequately with no health concerns, the nursing diagnoses are written with the focus of maintaining and protecting the client's health status. The nursing actions include support, praise, encouragement, dissemination of health information, and disease prevention. If the client has actual health problems, the client's strengths and wellness behaviors, actual or potential, are identified in conjunction with illness, diagnoses.

# How to Use
# This Handbook

## General Applications

This handbook is intended for use by nurses and other health care professionals whose objectives are health promotion and protection for their clients. It is assumed that the data-gathering phase of the process will be comprehensive and accurate. The nurse is then directed to the Nursing Diagnosis List grouped according to functional health patterns in this section. Having determined the nursing diagnosis category applicable to the client situation, the reader should proceed to Section II of this handbook. This section is organized according to functional health patterns. Each diagnostic category is defined and each nursing diagnosis statement is described in two parts. Health Status is identified as Part I of the Nursing Diagnosis Statement. Contributing Factors are then chosen as they best describe the circumstances of the client's health status. This becomes Part II of the Nursing Diagnosis—that follows the phrase "related to." The nurse then utilizes this wellness-oriented nursing diagnosis to determine interventions that develop, maintain, or enhance sound health practices or behaviors. Defining characteristics are written for each diagnosis that identifies observable data to support the diagnosis statement.

A list of commonly identified factors that contribute to wellness should be used as a reference point for the nurse to ensure a nursing diagnosis statement that is comprehensive and accurate (see box, Examples of Cues and Inferences). The nurse should thus use Section II to identify a specific contributing factor and she should also refer back to the box, Commonly Identified Factors That Contribute to Wellness, to establish the applicability of these commonly noted behaviors to the particular situation or circumstance of the client.

## Case Studies and Model Care Plans Using Wellness-Oriented Nursing Diagnoses

The final section of this handbook contains case studies and individualized care plans designed to illustrate the use of wellness-oriented nursing diagnoses. The examples were developed to assist the nurse, whose practice is holistic, in the analysis of assessment data for care planning that includes the identification of strengths or healthy behaviors present at some level in all persons. The case studies describe individual or family situations commonly encountered by the nurse in a variety of settings.

*Text continues on page 49*

## EXAMPLES OF CUES AND INFERENCES

### Subjective data

"I can't follow that diet it's too restrictive."

| *Cue* | *Inference* |
|---|---|
| Unable or unwilling to follow diet | Client is uncooperative. |

### Subjective Data

"I'm fearful of my husband's ability to cope with his illness."

| *Cue* | *Inference* |
|---|---|
| Expressed concern on the part of significant other | Client is unable or incapable of coping effectively. |

### Subjective Data

"But mom, all the kids at my school drink beer."

| *Cue* | *Inference* |
|---|---|
| Need for social acceptance | Epidemic of alcoholism among students |

### Subjective Data

"I try to get at least 8 hours of sleep every night."

| *Cue* | *Inference* |
|---|---|
| Awareness of the importance of the need for sleep | Client is well-rested. Client is compulsive regarding sleep needs. |

### Subjective Data

"I always take my pulse before and after my daily 3-mile run."

| *Cue* | *Inference* |
|---|---|
| Client verbalizes correlation between cardiovascular functioning and exercise. | Client is physically fit. Client is knowledgable regarding cardiovascular effects of aerobic exercise. Client is addicted to exercise regime. |

### Subjective data

"My mommy can't come to my school field trips because she works."

continued

| Cue | Inference |
|---|---|
| Child is stating a perception. | Mother uninterested in child's activities. Child is neglected. |

## Objective data

Mother: gravida V, para V, 1 day postpartum.

| Cue | Inference |
|---|---|
| Previous experience with childbirth/ childrearing. | Client has effective parenting skills. Client has a good knowledge base regarding newborn care. |

## Objective Data

Female: Height 5' 5"; weight 126 lbs

| Cue | Inference |
|---|---|
| Average height and weight | Good nutritional habits Regular exercise regime |

## Objective Data

Female, 32 years old, presents with a protuberant abdomen.

| Cue | Inference |
|---|---|
| Enlarged and distended abdomen | Client is pregnant. Client is obese. Client is an alcoholic. |

## Objective Data

Client is "sniffing."

| Cue | Inference |
|---|---|
| Client has rhinorrhea. | Client has allergies. Client has hayfever. Client is a cocaine addict. |

## Objective Data

Client looks at the floor frequently during the interview.

continued

| *Cue* | *Inference* |
|---|---|
| Client does not maintain eye contact. | Client is uninterested. Client is mistrustful. Client has a problem with sun-glare. |

**Objective Data**

Father slaps child's hand when he touches the otoscope.

| *Cue* | *Inference* |
|---|---|
| Father uses physical punishment to limit child's actions. | Child is abused. Father is concerned about discipline. Father is violent. |

**Objective Data**

Dirty dishes are stacked on the table and in the kitchen sink.

| *Cue* | *Inference* |
|---|---|
| Unwashed dishes | Hygiene deficit Slovenly housekeeper Potential for rodent infestation |

Although the examples are selective, they include the following circumstances: primary care settings, disease and trauma requiring hospitalization, terminal illness, health-risk appraisal, and growth and developmental issues for health promotion and protection in secondary and community health settings.

The individualized care plans have been developed utilizing the information contained in the case studies. As with the traditional nursing *analysis of assessment* data to identify problems, the past history and current health status of the individual or family described in the case study has been additionally analyzed for positive aspects of functioning. These positive aspects or strengths are either defining characteristics that actualize the strength or contributing factors that indicate the potential for positive health functioning.

The *wellness-oriented nursing diagnosis statements*, central to the care plans, were selected from the comprehensive list of possibilities included in this handbook. The traditional mode of functional health pattern identification followed by a review of possible associated nursing diagnoses has been utilized in these care planning examples to ensure congruence with the concept of the professional nursing process.

*Client-centered goals* are written in the traditional manner of the nursing process. The goal statements in the care plans indicate the desired outcomes of nursing care. It is interesting to note that long-and short-term goals are walkways defined in positive terms; that is, the identification of realistic and attainable outcomes, in collaboration with the client, that are at once positive and congruently supportive of client's needs. The development of goal statements for the model care plans further evidenced the need for a wellness-oriented nursing diagnosis. What better way is there to achieve positive outcomes than to identify the ways in which an individual or family has or can contribute to responsible self-care and healthy functioning?

The *nursing interventions* included in the care plans have also a positive orientation to ensure goal achievement. They are designed to capitalize on the identified strengths that are described in the nursing diagnosis statement. The nursing orders are written to incorporate the noted desires, skills, competencies, and developmental achievements of the individuals and families described in the case studies. The nursing actions have been individualized to the case study but they contain elements of health promotion and protection applicable to all consumers of nursing care services.

The *evaluative statements* included in the care plans define the terminal behaviors or outcome criteria indicative of goal achievement. These are written as statements of progression toward goal attainment, further development of identified strengths or growth toward responsible self-care.

The case studies do include information applicable to the identification of problems. The reader is directed to the list of problem-oriented nursing diagnoses in the box, Approved Nursing Diagnoses (North American Nursing Diagnosis Association, April 1986) and to the many excellent nursing processes texts that describe illness-related nursing diagnoses. Actual and potential problem identification has not been included in the care plans because the focus of this handbook is on the identification of wellness behaviors. These case studies and care plans are included for the purpose of facilitating the understanding of strength identification as an integral part of holistic nursing practice and to encourage the use of wellness-oriented nursing diagnoses in care planning.

# II

# Wellness-Oriented Nursing Diagnoses Grouped by Functional Health Patterns

## Functional Pattern 1:
# Health Perception—
# Health Management

### Health Maintenance

**Definition**

State in which an individual experiences or has the potential to experience a state of wellness because of adequate preventive measures or a healthy lifestyle.

**Nursing Diagnosis Statement**

*A. Health Status*

    Health maintenance, appropriate

*Text continues on page 66*

## Primary and Secondary Prevention for Age-Related Conditions

| DEVELOPMENTAL LEVEL | PRIMARY PREVENTION | SECONDARY PREVENTION |
| --- | --- | --- |
| Infancy (0–1 yrs) | Parent education<br>  Infant safety<br>  Nutrition<br>  Breast feeding<br>Sensory stimulation<br>  Infant massage and touch<br>  Visual stimulation<br>    Activity<br>    Colors<br>  Auditory stimulation<br>    Verbal<br>    Music<br>Immunizations<br>  DPT*<br>  TOPV*<br>Oral hygiene<br>  Teething biscuits<br>  Fluoride<br>  Avoid sugared food and drink | Complete physical exam every 2–3 months<br>Screening at birth<br>  Congenital hip<br>  Phenylketonuria<br>  Sickle cell<br>  Cystic fibrosis<br>  Vision (startle reflex)<br>  Hearing (response to and localization of sounds)<br>  TB test at 12 months<br>  Developmental assessments<br>Screen and intervene for high risk<br>  Low birth weight<br>  Maternal substance abuse during pregnancy |

## Primary and Secondary Prevention for Age-Related Conditions (continued)

| DEVELOPMENTAL LEVEL | PRIMARY PREVENTION | SECONDARY PREVENTION |
|---|---|---|
| | | Alcohol: fetal alcohol syndrome Cigarettes: SIDS Drugs: addicted neonate |
| | | Maternal infections during pregnancy |
| Preschool (1–5 yrs) | Parent education Teething Discipline Nutrition Accident prevention Normal growth and development Child education Dental self-care Dressing Bathing with assistance Feeding self-care | Complete physical exam between 2 and 3 years and preschool (U/A, CBC) TB test at 3 years Developmental assessments (annual) Speech development Hearing Vision Screen and intervene |

continued

## Primary and Secondary Prevention for Age-Related Conditions (continued)

| DEVELOPMENTAL LEVEL | PRIMARY PREVENTION | SECONDARY PREVENTION |
|---|---|---|
| | Immunizations<br>    DPT†<br>    TOPV†<br>    MMR at 15 months<br>Dental/oral hygiene<br>    Fluoride treatments<br>    Fluoridated water<br>Dietary counsel | Plumvism<br>    Developmental lag<br>    Neglect or abuse<br>    Strabismus<br>    Hearing deficit<br>    Vision deficit |
| School age (6–11 yrs) | Health education of child<br>    "Basic 4" nutrition<br>    Accident prevention<br>    Outdoor safety<br>    Substance abuse counsel<br>    Anticipatory guidance for physical changes at puberty<br>Immunizations<br>    Tetanus at age 10<br>    DPT‡<br>    TOPV‡<br>Dental hygiene every 6–12 months | Complete physical exam<br>    TB test every 3 years (at ages 6 and 9)<br>Developmental assessments<br>    Language<br>    Vision: Snellen charts at school<br>        6–8 years, use "E" chart<br>        Over 8 years, use alphabet chart |

## *Primary and Secondary Prevention for Age-Related Conditions (continued)*

| DEVELOPMENTAL LEVEL | PRIMARY PREVENTION | SECONDARY PREVENTION |
| --- | --- | --- |
| | | Hearing: audiogram |
| | Continue fluoridation Complete physical exam | |
| Adolescence (12–19 yrs) | Health education Proper nutrition and healthful diets Sex education with family planning, male/female Safe driving skills Adult challenges Seeking employment and career choices Dating and marriage Confrontation with substance abuse Safety in athletics Skin care Dental hygiene every 6–12 months | Complete physical exam (prepuberty or age 13) Blood pressure Cholesterol TB test at 12 years VDRL, CBC, U/A Female: breast self-exam (BSE) Male: testicular self-exam (TSE) Female, if sexually active: Pap and pelvic exam twice, 1 year apart (cervical gonorrhea culture |

continued

## Primary and Secondary Prevention for Age-Related Conditions (continued)

| DEVELOPMENTAL LEVEL | PRIMARY PREVENTION | SECONDARY PREVENTION |
|---|---|---|
| | Immunizations<br>  Tetanus without<br>  trauma<br>  TOPV booster at<br>  12–14 years | with pelvic); then every 3 years if both are negative<br>Screening and interventions<br>  Depression<br>  Suicide<br>  Substance abuse<br>  Pregnancy (more than 18 years old)<br>  Family history of alcoholism or domestic violence |
| Young adult (20–39 yrs) | Health education<br>Weight management with good nutrition as BMR changes<br>Life-style counseling<br>  Stress management<br>  Safe driving<br>  Family<br>  Parenting skills<br>  Regular exercise<br>  Environmental health choices | Complete physical exam at about 20 years, then every 5–6 years<br>Cancer checkup every 3 years<br>Female: BSE monthly<br>Male: TSE monthly<br>All females: baseline mammography |

## *Primary and Secondary Prevention for Age-Related Conditions (continued)*

| DEVELOPMENTAL LEVEL | PRIMARY PREVENTION | SECONDARY PREVENTION |
|---|---|---|
| | Dental hygiene every 6–12 months<br><br>Immunization<br>    Tetanus at 20 years and every 10 years<br>    Female: rubella, if zero negative for antibodies | between ages 35 and 40<br><br>Parents-to-be: high-risk screening for Down syndrome, Tay–Sachs<br><br>Female pregnant: screen for VD, rubella titer, Rh factor<br><br>Screening and interventions if high risk<br>    Female with previous breast cancer: Annual mammography at 35 years and after<br>    Female with mother or sister who has had breast cancer (same as above)<br>    Family history colorectal cancer |

continued

## Primary and Secondary Prevention for Age-Related Conditions (continued)

| DEVELOPMENTAL LEVEL | PRIMARY PREVENTION | SECONDARY PREVENTION |
|---|---|---|
| | | or high risk: Annual stool guaiac, digital, rectal, and sigmoidoscopy PPD if exposed to TB |
| Middle-aged adult (40–59 yrs) | Health education: continue with young adult | Complete physical exam every 5–6 years with complete laboratory evaluation (serum/urine tests, x-ray, ECG) |
| | Midlife changes, male and female counseling "Empty-nest" syndrome Anticipatory guidance Grandparenting | Cancer checkup every year |
| | Dental hygiene every 6–12 months | Female: BSE monthly |
| | Immunizations Tetanus every 10 years | Male: TSE monthly |
| | Pneumococcal: annual if high risk, *i.e.*, major chronic disease (COPD, CAD) | All females: annual mammography 50 years and over |
| | | Schiotz' tonometry (glaucoma) every 3–5 years |

## *Primary and Secondary Prevention for Age-Related Conditions (continued)*

| DEVELOPMENTAL LEVEL | PRIMARY PREVENTION | SECONDARY PREVENTION |
|---|---|---|
| | Influenza (same as above) | Female pregnant: prenatal screening by amniocentesis or chorionic villus sampling, if desired. |
| | | Sigmoidoscopy at ages 50 and 51, then every 4 years if negative |
| | | Stool guaiac annually at age 50 and thereafter |
| | | Screening and intervention if high risk<br>Endometrial cancer: Have endometrial sampling at menopause<br>Oral cancer: Screen more often if substance abuser |
| Elderly adult (60–74 yrs) | Health education: continue with previous | Complete physical exam every 2 years |

continued

*Primary and Secondary Prevention for Age-Related Conditions (continued)*

| DEVELOPMENTAL LEVEL | PRIMARY PREVENTION | SECONDARY PREVENTION |
|---|---|---|
| | counseling | with laboratory assessments |
| | Home safety | Annual cancer checkup |
| | Retirement | Blood pressure annually |
| | Loss of spouse | Female: BSE monthly |
| | Special health needs | Male: TSE monthly |
| | Nutritional changes | Female: annual mammogram |
| | Changes in hearing or vision | Annual stool guaiac |
| | Alterations in bowel or bladder habits | Sigmoidoscopy every 4 years |
| | Dental/oral hygiene every 6–12 months | Schiotz' tonometry every 3–5 years |
| | Immunizations | Podiatric evaluation with food care prn |
| | Tetanus every 10 years | Screen for high risk |
| | Pneumococcal§ | Depression |
| | Influenza§ | Suicide |
| Old-aged adult (75 yrs +) | Complete physical exam annually | Health education: Continue counsel |

## Primary and Secondary Prevention for Age-Related Conditions (continued)

| DEVELOPMENTAL LEVEL | PRIMARY PREVENTION | SECONDARY PREVENTION |
|---|---|---|
| | Laboratory assessments | Anticipatory guidance |
| | Cancer checkup | Dying and death |
| | Blood pressure | Loss of spouse |
| | Stool guaiac | Increasing dependency on others |
| | Female: mammogram, sigmoidoscopy every 4 years | Dental/oral hygiene every 6–12 months |
| | Schiotz' tonometry every 3–5 years | Immunizations |
| | Podiatrist prn | Tetanus every 10 years |
| | | Pneumococcal‖ |
| | | Influenza‖ |

*At 2, 3, and 6 months.
†At 18 months.
‡Boosters between 4 and 6 years.
§Annual if high risk.
‖Annually.
BMR = basal metabolic rate; BSE = breast self-examination; CBC = complete blood count; DPT = diphtheria-pertussis-tetanus; ECG = electrocardiogram; MMR = measles, mumps, rubella; PPD = purified protein derivative; prn = as circumstances may require; TB = tuberculosis; TOPV = trivalent oral polio virus vaccine; TSE = testes self-examination; U/A = urinalysis; VD = venereal disease; VDRL = Venereal Disease Research Laboratories.
(Adapted from Carpenito LJ: Handbook of Nursing Diagnosis. Philadelphia, JB Lippincott, 1984)

### B. *Contributing Factors*

Balanced rest/activity pattern
Accessibility to health care services
Internal locus of control
Age-appropriate supervision for children
Good oral hygiene
Regular physical examinations/dental
Adequate prenatal care
Normal birth weight
Regular physical examinations
Normal growth and development
Adequate health practices
Nutritional diet
Reasonable weight management
Weight management with good nutrition
Regular exercise regime
Good parenting skills
Awareness (practice) of home safety
Supportive environment

## C. Defining Characteristics

Appropriate health promotion/protection
   activities
Up-to-date immunization schedule
Regular exercise program
Cleanliness
Routine dental care
Routine physical examinations
Adequate diet
Good muscle tone
Appropriate energy level
Emotional stability

---

## Accident Prevention

### Definition

The approach to daily living that minimizes potential and actual threats of bodily harm.

## Nursing Diagnosis Statement

### A. Health Status

Accident prevention practices, adequate (to support personal safety)

Hazard management, effective (to prevent injury)

Safety practices, satisfactory (to manage potential problems)

Potential for practice of adequate safety precautions

### B. Contributing Factors

Evidence of effective management of safety in activities of daily living

Use of safety restraints while traveling

Awareness of factors with potential for injuries/accidents

Awareness of unhealthy and unsafe practices

Physical capabilities for activities supporting health and safe life-style

Effective life-style management (time, priorities)

Appropriate use of over-the-counter or prescribed medications (with effects or side effects related to judgment, lethargy, and diminished reaction time)

Judicious use of alcohol

Support of available significant other(s) regarding safety awareness and safety practices in daily activities

## C. *Defining Characteristics*

Absence of injury

Focus on safety awareness

# Functional Pattern 2:
# *Nutrition—Metabolic*

## *Nutrition*

### Definition

The processes by which the body receives and utilizes nutrients to provide energy, build and maintain body tissues, and regulate metabolic reactions required for the activities of daily living.

### Nursing Diagnosis Statement

#### A. *Health Status*

Nutritional status, optimal

Nutrition, adequate to meet or maintain body requirements

Nutritional intake, effective for optimal growth

Potential for reaching satisfactory nutritional intake to meet metabolic needs

### B. Contributing Factors

Awareness of programs available to support good nutrition (*e.g.,* Women Infant Children program (WIC), Meals on Wheels)

Awareness and use of financial assistance (*e.g.,* food stamps)

Knowledge of special age- and sex-related nutritional needs

Understanding of rationale for dietary modifications

Evidence of appropriate balance between nutrition, activity, and elimination

Knowledge of interaction of medications and food/drink

Appropriate intake/use of alcohol, caffeine, refined sugars, salt, fats, additives, prescribed medications, and tobacco

Satisfying social, religious, or cultural practices

Availability of support from significant others

Appropriate management of nutritionally related problems

Ability to read and comprehend nutritional
information

Appropriately fitting dentures

Adequate oral hygiene

## C. Defining Characteristics

Adequate nutritional status

Weight within 10% of Ideal Body Weight for
height, build, age, and sex

Skinfold thickness not greater than one inch:
percentage of body fat not greater than
20% for females, 19% for males (adult
using 3–4 skinfold sites)

No fatty deposits/bulges

Energy level appropriately maintained

No physical evidence of nutritional deficit

(teeth, hair, skin, mucous membranes, and nails)

---

## *Fluid and Electrolytes*

### Definition

The nutrient substances that regulate specific body processes and whose levels need to be regulated to maintain homeostasis. These include water, sodium, potassium, magnesium, calcium, chloride, phosphorus, and bicarbonate.

### Nursing Diagnosis Statement

#### A. Health Status

Fluid volume, adequate to support bodily needs

Hydration status, optimal

Fluid exchange rate, adequate to meet metabolic requirements

Fluid intake, appropriate to support activities
of daily living
Potential for achieving satisfactory hydration
status to meet metabolic needs

**B. *Contributing Factors***

Intake appropriate to output
Appropriate protein intake
Adequate lymphatic drainage
Adequate cardiovascular functioning
Adequate renal function
Adequate liver function
Hormonal balance
Accurate and sufficient information relative to
sound hydration practices
Knowledge of the influence of exercise, tem-
perature, drugs, caffeine, and alcohol on
fluid balance: rationale for modification of
fluid and electrolyte intake
Availability of adequate resources to support
appropriate hydration (financial, location,

access, transfer, materials, and clean $H_2O$ supply)

Evidence of appropriate balance between activity, elimination, nutrition, and hydration

Appropriate management of problems related to hydration

Appropriate use of medications

Appropriate dietary régime

## C. Defining Characteristics

Good skin turgor

Moist mucous membranes

Adequate tear formation

Adequate urine production/elimination (adult 200 ml/hr 2000 ml/24°)

No evidence of sunken eyes or fontanels

No edema (pitting or dependent) ascites, anasarca, or hydrothorax

Absence of weakness, confusion, fatigue, oliguria, paresthesia, and fever

Urine specific gravity = 1.001–1.035 adult
  and child
Appropriate dietary sodium intake
No excessive thirst
Stable body weight
Afebrile state
Stool elimination regular and soft consistency

---

## *Immune Response*

### Definition

The defense function of the body that produces antibodies to destroy invading antigens and malignancies.

### Nursing Diagnosis Statement

#### *A. Health Status*

Immune response, effective

## B. Contributing Factors

Efficient phagocytic system
Intact integumentary system
Adequate inflammatory response
Resistance to infection
Low virulence of invading pathogens
Mental health
Proper diet
Healthful environment
Appropriate rest/activity balance
Efficient circulatory functioning
Antibody-mediated response
Cell-mediated response
Synergistic complement system
Age-appropriate immunizations

## C. Defining Characteristics

Minimal/no exposure to infectious diseases
Minimal episodes of infectious processes
Adherence to immunization schedule

Physical resources to cope and recover from
  infectious episodes
WBC within normal limits
Afebrile
Absence of lethargy and irritability
Negative culture and sensitivity as appropriate
Appropriate antibody screening results

---

## *Integumentary*

### Definition

The part of the body that functions as a physical
barrier between the internal body organs and the
environment. It consists of intact skin and mucous
membranes.

### Nursing Diagnosis Statement

#### *A. Health Status:*

Skin integrity, adequate (to support body
  requirements)

Integumentary status, effective (for support of optimal health)

Skin and mucous membrane status, optimal (to meet or maintain body needs)

Potential for satisfactory skin integrity to meet health maintenance needs

## B. *Contributing Factors*

Evidence of appropriate nutrition, hydration, rest, and hygiene practices

Awareness of factors that influence the status of the integumentary system (diet, hydration, sun exposure, stress, topical applications—creams, make-up, sun block, cleansers, and medications)

Knowledge of and effective practices for the care of individual skin conditions (acne, dry skin, moles, and cysts).

Awareness of significance of changes in existing long-standing skin lesions

Appropriate use of over-the-counter or prescribed medications for the maintenance of
integrity for integumentary system

Effective management of environmental factors influencing skin condition (light, heat,
humidity, circulating air, and dust/dirt)

## C. Defining Characteristics

Skin and mucous membranes intact

Decreased fragility

Good skin turgor

No edema, ecchymosis, abnormal growths

Minimal exposure to irritants

# Functional Pattern 3:
# *Elimination*

## *Bowel Elimination*

### Definition

The process by which the body rids itself of solid-waste products that were undigested or unabsorbed during the nutritional process. It involves the defecation of feces.

### Nursing Diagnosis Statement

#### A. Health Status

Bowel elimination, adequate

Bowel elimination, optimal (to support daily activities and comfort)

Bowel elimination, satisfactory (to support homeostasis)

Potential for establishing effective bowel elimination pattern to meet metabolic requirements and comfort

## B. *Contributing Factors*

Evidence of appropriate balance between nutrition, exercise, and elimination

Awareness of foods and substances that have laxative, constipating, or gas-producing effects

Adequate diet

Knowledge of significance of notable changes in bowel habits

Active (vs sedentary) life-style with effective management of changes in daily routines

Adequate fluid intake

Appropriate compensation for fluid losses related to environmental temperature and activity

Minimal use of over-the-counter or prescribed

medications for maintenance of regularity
or control of constipation or diarrhea
Awareness and effective nutritional compensa-
tion for medications producing constipating
or diarrhea-inducing effects or side effects
Effective intestinal functioning
Regular defecation pattern
Appropriate GI motility
Adequate sphincter reflexes
Support of available significant other(s) re-
garding positive bowel training habits, pri-
vacy, independence, and dignity.

## C. Defining Characteristics

Routine passage of stool
Appropriate color consistency, amount, and
odor of stool
Absence of rectal pain, abdominal discomfort,
fecal bloating impaction, nausea, or vomiting
Soft, nontender abdomen
Absence of constipation/diarrhea

> Negative hematest/guaiac stools
> Absence of pathology

---

## Bladder Elimination

### Definition

The process by which the body rids itself of water and electrolytes that are the metabolic end products of the nutrition process. It involves a complex series of events in which urine is formed in the kidney and passes through the ureters to the urinary bladder. Micturition of the urine then occurs.

### Nursing Diagnosis Statement

#### A. Health Status

   Bladder elimination, adequate
   Urinary elimination, optimal (to support homeostasis)
   Bladder elimination, satisfactory (to support body needs and comfort)

Potential for effective urinary elimination
pattern

**B. *Contributing Factors***

Evidence of appropriate balance between fluid
intake and urinary elimination (good skin
turgor, moist mucous membranes, and absence of edema)

Awareness of fluids and foods that enhance or
diminish urinary elimination

Knowledge of significance of notable changes
in bladder habits

Effective life-style management (stress,
changes in routine)

Adequate fluid intake with appropriate compensation for fluid losses related to environmental temperature or perspiration

Efficient renal functioning

Appropriate use of over-the-counter or prescribed medications (for the maintenance
of urinary output and the prevention of
fluid retention)

Awareness of effective nutritional and fluid intake compensation for medications affecting urinary output

Effective hygiene practices related to urinary elimination

Support of available significant other(s) (regarding positive bladder training habits, privacy, independence, and dignity)

Comfort level adequate to support the establishment of a healthy pattern of urinary elimination

## C. Defining Characteristics

Unobstructed passage of urine

Amount consistent with intake

Urinalysis within normal limits

Clear, pale yellow urine

Absence of sediment and/or froth

Absence of foul-smelling or fruity odor

Negative urine culture

# *Functional Pattern 4:*
# *Activity—Exercise*

## *Mobility*

### Definition

The process by which the body utilizes motion to accomplish activities of daily living, to assist in the maintenance of bodily functions, and to achieve physical fitness.

### Nursing Diagnosis Statement

### A. *Health Status*

Activity tolerance

Optimal physical fitness

Mobility level, adequate (to meet demands of daily living)

Activity level, adequate (to support body maintenance)

Exercise level, appropriate (to maintain wellness state)

Potential for achieving optimal physical fitness and activity level

## B. *Contributing Factors*

Evidence of appropriate balance between nutrition, rest, and mobility

Awareness of effective nutrition, fluid, and rest compensation for healthy balance and activity

Knowledge and practice of appropriate safety measures (to support healthy activity practices)

Integration of exercise regimen with life-style/role responsibilities

Appropriate use and management of over-the-counter or prescribed medications

Comfort level adequate (to support the estab-
   lishment of a health pattern of mobility)
Effective management of factors interfering
   with the ability to maintain activity
Support of significant other(s) (regarding the
   establishment and maintenance of health
   activity patterns)
Age-appropriate development
Functional musculoskeletal system
Appropriate sensory ability and proprioception
Adequate cardiovascular functioning
Adequate respiratory functioning
Sense of industry

## C. Defining Characteristics

Evidence of flexibility, agility, and endurance
Cardiorespiratory endurance
Muscular strength/endurance
Achievement/maintenance of developmental
   motor skills

## *Respiratory Function*

### Definition

The state in which the individual experiences the passage of air through the respiratory tract and an exchange of gases ($O_2$, $CO_2$) between the lungs and the vascular system.

### Nursing Diagnosis Statement

*A. Health Status*

Respiratory function, effective

*B. Contributing Factors*

Normal blood gases

Efficient cough reflex

Adequate cardiac/respiratory functioning

Normal pulmonary artery/right ventricular pressure

Adequate neuromuscular functioning

Appropriate lung elasticity

Healthy lung tissue

Appropriate anatomic structure

Ability to maintain demands of activities of
   daily living

Minimal environmental pollution

Minimal/no use of inhalants

Normal lung compliance

## C. *Defining Characteristics*

Symmetrical expansion of chest

Appropriate depth of respiration

Appropriate rate of respiration

Appropriate pattern of respiration

Adequate oxygenation

Clear breath sounds

Adequate coping mechanisms

Effective mucous clearance

Appropriate skin color

## *Cardiac Function*

### Definition

Adequate cardiac output due to the ability of the heart to effectively pump and circulate the blood supply.

### Nursing Diagnosis Statement

#### A. *Health Status*

Cardiac functioning, effective

#### B. *Contributing Factors*

Normal stroke volume
Normal blood pressure readings
Vascular sufficiency/patency
Appropriate pulmonary functioning
Fluid and electrolyte balance
Appropriate management of stress
Appropriate anatomic structure

Proper rest–activity/exercise balance
Proper medication administration
Proper dietary régime
Adequate respiratory/cardiac functioning

## C. *Defining Characteristics*

Appropriate cardiac rate/rhythm
Adequate cardiac cycle
Effective conduction system
Valvular sufficiency
Absence of pain/discomfort and signs of associated cardiorespiratory symptomatology

---

# Home Maintenance Management

## Definition

The state in which an individual or family has the ability or the potential ability, to maintain self or family in a safe home environment.

## Nursing Diagnosis Statement

### A. Health Status

Home maintenance management, effective

### B. Contributing Factors

Ability to cope with illness or injury to an individual or family member

Appropriate cognitive processing

Sufficient resources (financial, psychological, educational, and physical)

Proper hygienic practices

Appropriate motivation of caregivers

Proper storage and disposal of hazardous substances

### C. Defining Characteristics

Maintenance of household

Adequate individual/family coping patterns

Knowledgeable caregiver

## Self-Care Ability

### Definition

The state in which an individual is able to feed, bathe, dress, or toilet oneself.

### Nursing Diagnosis Statement

*A. Health Status*

Self-care, independence

*B. Contributing Factors*

Appropriate coordination

Normal musculoskeletal functioning

Appropriate neuromuscular functioning

Appropriate sensory functioning

Effective cognitive processing

High motivational level

Need for independence

Ability to effectively cope with a disability
(specify)

Effective health maintenance program
Age-appropriate development
Supportive environment
Accommodating physical environment

### C. Defining Characteristics

Adequate knowledge base
Independence in feeding, bathing, grooming, dressing, and toileting

## Functional Pattern 5:
# Sleep—Rest

### Sleep Pattern

#### Definition

A complex biological rhythm consisting of four stages during which the body relaxes and is restored physically and mentally. This offsets the fatigue induced by the activities of daily living.

#### Nursing Diagnosis Statement

*A. Health Status*

Sleep pattern, adequate (to meet demands of daily living)

Sleep and rest periods, effective (for healthy bodily maintenance)

Sleep quality, duration, and frequency appropriate to support wellness

Potential for achieving optimally effective sleep/rest pattern

## B. *Contributing Factors*

Evidence of appropriate balance between rest/sleep and activity

Physical and mental capability to fall asleep and maintain adequate restful sleep periods (or effective management of disabilities)

Awareness of factors that induce and inhibit sleep and rest

Effective life-style management (stress, travel)

Adequate comfort level

Appropriate use of over-the-counter or prescribed medications that affect sleep patterns and rest periods

Effective management of environmental stimuli affecting rest/sleep (noise, light, and temperature)

Support of available significant other(s) related
    to the establishment and maintenance of
    healthy sleep/rest patterns
Effective use of safety precautions related to
    sleep areas
Ability to adjust to interruptions in usual sleep
    patterns

## C. *Defining Characteristics*

Attentive to daytime activities
Hours of sleep adequate for age/stage of
    development
Established bedtime routine/rituals
Reports of sufficient energy for activities of
    daily living

# Functional Pattern 6:
# *Cognitive—Perceptual*

## *Developmental Growth*

(Including that of exceptional individuals)

### Definition

Development is a continuous evolutionary process that proceeds in the direction of increasing complexity and diversity. Each person's development is a unique process that emerges out of the individual's innate abilities and continuous interaction with the environment. An exceptional individual is a person whose growth or development deviates from the norm in some way. Traditionally, the term has been applied to retarded, disabled, or very bright children. This category includes, but is not limited to, the traditional definition as the statements are applicable to all persons in any state of development throughout the life span.

## Nursing Diagnosis Statement

### A. Health Status

Developmental progression, efficient

Potential for successful satisfaction of developmental needs

### B. Contributing Factors

Personal Factors

Realistic expectation of functioning

Willingness to explore alternative life-styles

Adaptive behavior

Adequate attention span

Desire to learn

Ability to form concepts and abstractions

Accurate perception of personal abilities

Adequate retention of information

Verbalization of emotions and feelings

Realistic future aspirations

Recognition and/or acceptance of limitations
or assets

Assumption of age or ability appropriate
responsibilities

Ability to achieve developmental tasks

Use of rehabilitative resources

Feeling of competence

Achievement of a sense of personal identity

Appropriate sexual identity

Problem-solving ability

Ability to initiate (maintain) friendships

Ability to make appropriate decisions


Parental Factors

Supportive parenting

Realistic expectation of functioning

Challenging intellectual environment

Encouragement of personal growth and
potential

Willingness to explore alternative life-styles

Consistent limit setting

Realistic future aspirations

Acceptance of limitations or assets

Parental support of child's special abilities

Opportunities to develop self-esteem or
independence

Realistic utilization of institutional care

Social Factors

Interpersonal relationships with potential for
growth

Realistic expectation of functioning

Challenging intellectual environment

Creative utilization of abilities

Encouragement of personal growth and
potential

Open expression of emotions and feelings

Appropriate use of remediation or enrichment
activities

Opportunities to develop self-esteem or
independence

Professional Factors

    Knowledgeable caregivers

    Realistic expectation of functioning

    Challenging intellectual environment

    Creative utilization of abilities

    Encouragement of personal growth and
       potential

    Willingness to explore alternative life-styles

    Consistent limit setting

    Realistic future aspirations

    Acceptance of limitations or assets

    Positive role models

    Nurturing relationships

    Opportunities to develop self-esteem or
       independence

## C. *Defining Characteristics*

    Progressive psychosexual/psychosocial
       development

    Achievement of developmental milestones at
       an appropriate pace

## *Comfort*

### Definition

The state in which the body is relieved of unpleasant sensory or environmental stimuli.

### Nursing Diagnosis Statement

#### A. Health Status

Comfort, adequate

Potential for comfort

#### B. Contributing Factors

Proper body alignment

Effective safety measures

Effective medication management

Appropriate therapeutic management

Mental health

External temperature regulation

Use of relaxation techniques

Appropriate rest/activity balance
Supportive environment

## C. *Defining Characteristics*
Adequate need satisfaction
Feeling of well-being

---

## *Sensory Functioning*

### Definition

Visual, auditory, olfactory, gustatory, and tactile ability are intact.

### Nursing Diagnosis Statement

#### A. *Health Status*
Sensory functioning (*e.g.*, visual), adequate
Potential for successful coping of diminished sensory ability (*e.g.*, auditory)

## B. *Contributing Factors*

Preventive health maintenance practices

Use of appropriate safety measures

Acceptance (use) of necessary auxilliary
devices

Acceptance of limitations

Integration of limitations into life-style

Appropriate therapeutic management

Effective teaching/learning activities

Prompt and effective treatment of illnesses
(*e.g.,* otitis media)

## C. *Defining Characteristics*

Intact sensory functioning

# Functional Pattern 7:
## *Self-Perception*

## *Adaptive Stress Response (Anxiety)*

### Definition

A state in which the individual is motivated to action as a result of the feeling of apprehension and activation initiated by the autonomic nervous system's response to a vague, nonspecific threat.

### Nursing Diagnosis Statement

#### A. Health Status

Stress response, adaptive

Potential for resolution of personal threat

### B. Contributing Factors

Supportive Network

    Willingness to try new coping skills

    Realistic perception of the situation

    Adequate coping mechanisms

    Productive problem-solving ability

    Realistic personal expectations

    Balance in rest and activity patterns

    Understanding of personal response to stress

    Successful coping with prior stressors

    Anticipating and preparing for change

    Realistic identification of contributing factors

    Ability to utilize more effective coping skills

    Understanding the relationship between anxiety and the precipitating event

    Ability to evaluate personal coping style

    Awareness of the effect of anxiety on personal behavior and life-style

    Identification of current events as related to past experiences

    Successful defense system

## C. *Defining Characteristics*

Increased alertness

Focus on problem

Stimulation of sympathetic stress system
  (fight-or-flight response)

Established plan of action

---

# *Self-Concept*

## Definition

All the notions, beliefs, and convictions that constitute an individual's knowledge of self and influence his relationships with others.

## Nursing Diagnosis Statement

### A. *Health Status*

Self-concept, positive

**B. *Contributing Factors***

Appropriate self-expectation

Ability to initiate and maintain intimate relationships

Appropriate understanding and integration of childhood experiences

Discriminating sense of trust

Appropriate psychosocial development

Successful developmental task mastery

Appropriate impulse control

Development of internal moral judgment

Ability to compete appropriately with others

Establishment of realistic life goals

Effective personal integration

Healthy ego development

Appropriate sense of (emerging) personal identity

Ability to cope effectively with stressors (change, loss, crisis, death)

Ability to adapt to changing family configurations

Ability to cope with altered living
   arrangements
Appropriate care and stimulation during in-
   fancy and childhood
Ability to adapt to maturational changes
Internal locus of control
Satisfying peer relationships

## C. Defining Characteristics
Achievement of goals
Adaptability
Subjective statement of feelings of well-being

---

## Body Image

### Definition

The mental representation of one's body derived
from internal sensations, emotions, fantasies, pos-
ture, and experience of and with external objects
and people.

**Nursing Diagnosis Statement**

*A. Health Status*

Body image, positive

Body image, realistic

*B. Contributing Factors*

Acceptance of disability

Maturational awareness of separateness of own body

Appropriate perception of body boundary

Adaptation to maturational changes of body boundary

Appropriate differentiation of self

Integrity of perceptual systems

Adaptation to disability

Appropriate somatosensory stimulation

Nurturing caregiving activities during infancy and childhood

Appropriate stimulation and play activities during infancy and childhood

Coping with deformity, disfigurement, or
   disease
Acceptance of rehabilitation needs
Appropriate strategies to seek and direct own
   medical treatment
Ability to estimate relationship of body to
   environment
Personal acceptance by significant others
Appropriate peer identification/peer
   acceptance
Congruence of personal and sociocultural
   attitudes
Understanding of media influence

## C. Defining Characteristics

Positive reinforcement from significant others
Ability to touch or look at a diseased or dis-
   figured body part

## *Self-Esteem*

### Definition

The degree to which one feels valued, worthwhile, or competent.

### Nursing Diagnosis Statement

#### A. *Health Status*

Self-esteem, positive

#### B. *Contributing Cognitive Factors*

Self-acceptance
Appreciation of the unique value of oneself
Recognition (acceptance) of one's limitations
Holistic recognition (acceptance) of one's
   qualities
Recognition (acceptance) of one's strengths
Recognition (acceptance) of one's accomplish-
   ments/failures

Acceptance of maturational changes

Coping with changes in self as a result of maturation, illness, accident, or disfigurement

Healthy relationships with others

Congruence of sociocultural expectations

Affective Factors

Effective tension-relieving behaviors

Ability to verbalize feelings

Appropriate expression of feelings and emotions

Spiritual strength

Assertive behavior

Physiologic Factors

Increased alertness

Use of relaxation techniques

Proper health habits

Physical stamina

Social Factors

Seeking (accepting) help from others

### C. Defining Characteristics
Successful parenting
(see Self-Concept category for other
characteristics)

# Functional Pattern 8:
# Role—Relationship

(Family Interactions, Social Relationships)

## Effective Family Coping

### Definition

The state in which a family demonstrates constructive behaviors associated with the ability to manage internal and external stressors due to adequate physical, psychosocial, and cognitive resources.

### Nursing Diagnosis Statement

#### A. Health Status

Coping, effective family
Family processes, productive
Family functioning, satisfactory

## B. *Contributing Factors*

Parental Factors

- Consensual decision making
- Acceptance of expression of feeling and emotions
- Family unity
- Role flexibility
- Open communication patterns
- Encouragement of personal growth and potential
- Respect for individuality of family members
- Constructive discipline practices
- Attention to unique emotional needs of each of the family members
- Adequate provision of food and shelter
- Appropriate management of space
- Physical health of family members
- Acceptance of reality regarding individual health problems
- Sensitivity to family member's needs

Sufficient satisfaction from sexual relations

Spiritual strength

Recognition of individual accomplishments

Acceptance of personal problems

Open expression of affection

Ethical value framework

Sufficient encouragement of each other's efforts

Provision for recreation

Positive identification of child's (children's) individual characteristics

Availability of family members

Appropriate distribution of responsibilities

Balance in family activity patterns

Self-realization of parents

Seeking (accepting) help when needed

Ability to use a crisis constructively

Intrafamily cooperation

Realistic expectations of one another

Attention to one another's physical and psychosocial needs

Acceptance of personal responsibility

Ability to meet responsibility

Sibling Factors

Acceptance of expression of feelings and emotions

Family unity

Respect for individuality of family members

Physical health of family members

Acceptance of reality regarding individual health problems

Sensitivity to each other's needs

Recognition of individual accomplishments

Acceptance of personal problems

Open expression of affection

Ethical value framework

Sufficient encouragement of each other's efforts

Provision for recreation

Participation in family activities
Balance in family activity patterns
Seeking (accepting) help when needed
Ability to use a crisis constructively
Intrafamily cooperation
Realistic expectations of one another
Attention to one another's physical and psychosocial needs
Respect for parents/authority
Supportive sibling relationships
Acceptance of personal responsibility
Ability to meet responsibility

Extended Family Factors
Fulfilling intergenerational relationships
Open communication patterns

Social Factors
Membership in social organizations
Initiation and maintenance of individual friendships and relationships
Growthful relationships

### C. Defining Characteristics

Adequate family coping patterns

Open communication patterns

Responsible childrearing practices: limit-setting, nurturance

---

## Satisfying Social Interactions

### Definition

The state in which an individual experiences a productive social interaction with the ability to experience pleasure and to resolve conflicts constructively.

### Nursing Diagnosis Statement

### A. Health Status

Social interaction, satisfactory

Social functioning, productive

**B. *Contributing Factors***

Personal Factors

    Feelings of usefulness

    Independent thinking

    Acceptance (recognition) of individuality

    Ability to make decisions

    Seeking (accepting) companionship with others

    High energy level

    Interest in a variety of activities

    Constructive management of stressors

    Sound judgment

    Ability to meet responsibilities

    Personal maturity

    Constructive resolution of conflicts

    Realistic belief about self-worth

    Recognition of self-worth and abilities

Social Factors

    Ability to initiate activities

Experiences of pleasure
Ability to form and maintain relationships
Respect for others
Desire to give to others
Ability to recognize trustworthy individuals
Ability to trust others
Understanding of (respect for) social norms
Ability to meet responsibilities
Work (school) satisfaction
Constructive resolution of conflicts
Ability to resolve conflicting loyalties and philosophies of life
Respect for authority
Ability to establish intimacy
Ability to accept the limitations of others
Ability to support others
Ability to meet role expectations
Ability to adapt to a new environment (work, school)

## C. Defining Characteristics
   Trustworthiness
   Adaptability

# Functional Pattern 9:
# *Sexuality—Reproductive*

## *Satisfactory Sexual Functioning*

### Definition

The state in which an individual experiences satisfaction with gender, sex role, and behaviors associated with one's chosen sexual identity and activities. Satisfactory sexual functioning contributes to the personal health and well-being of oneself and others.

### Nursing Diagnosis Statement

#### A. Health Status

Sexual function, adequate

Sexual expression, appropriate

Gender identity, appropriate
Sexual activities, satisfactory

## B. Contributing Factors

Personal Factors

Adaptation to changes associated with aging, disease, surgery, and role transitions

Adaptation to changes associated with childbearing

Recognition (acceptance) of self as sexual being

Effective management of feelings of developing sexuality

Ability to communicate sexual needs

Ability to experience intimacy

Value clarification skills

Responsibility for sexual behavior

Congruity with personal value system

Interest in a variety of activities

Responsibility for conception control

Age appropriate psychosexual development

Social Factors

Effective role models

Availability of correct information about
sexuality

Resolution of value conflicts associated with
sexual expression

Healthy relationship with significant other

Experience of pleasure from sexual activities

### C. *Defining Characteristics*

Satisfaction with sex role, gender

Adequate sexual performance

Adequate knowledge base

Reports sexual satisfaction

# Functional Pattern 10:
## Coping—Stress Tolerance

### Crisis Resolution

#### Definition

The process of effective coping and resolution of a crisis and restoration to a level of functioning equal to, or better than, that of the precrisis level.

#### Nursing Diagnosis Statement

##### A. Health Status

Crisis resolution, effective
Potential for improved level of functioning

##### B. Contributing Factors

Appropriate coping mechanisms
Productive problem-solving ability

Seeking or accepting help when needed
Ability to meet role responsibilities
Correct health habits
Successful coping with a previous crisis
Appropriate expression of distress
Evidence of personal growth
Supportive network

### C. Defining Characteristics
Strong support system
Realistic perception of a situation
Open expression and acknowledgment of
    emotions

---

## Effective Individual Coping

### Definition

A state in which the individual demonstrates an
ability to manage internal, developmental, or exter-

nal stressors appropriately due to adequate physical, psychosocial, and cognitive resources.

## Nursing Diagnosis Statement

### A. Health Status

Coping, effective individual

Management of stressors, productive

### B. Contributing Factors

Personal Factors

Development of personal identity (age-appropriate)

Establishment of independence (age-appropriate)

Ability to control impulses (age-appropriate)

Ability to communicate effectively

Ability to problem-solve (age-appropriate)

Balance of activities

Decision-making ability (age-appropriate)

Appropriate expression of feelings and emotions

Physical health
Acceptance of reality of health problems
Adequate provision of food and shelter
Spiritual strength
Realistic perception of accomplishments
Realistic perception of deficiencies
Ethical value framework
Ability to use crisis constructively
Ability to meet role expectations
Successful arrival at next stage of
    development
Acceptance of a new role
Success with previous life transitions
Ability to accept responsibility for actions
Progression through the stages of grief and
    mourning

Social Factors
Successful adaptation to a new environment
    (school, work)

Positive work (school) adjustment

Seeking support systems

Growthful interpersonal relationships

Supportive family relationships

Adequate social network

Participation in social organizations

Sufficient satisfaction from sexual relations

Adequate role models

## C. *Defining Characteristics*

Basic human needs satisfied

Acknowledgment and expression of feelings

# Functional Pattern 11:
## Spiritual Support

---

## Spirituality

### Definition

The state in which the individual experiences comfort in his beliefs or value system which is his source of strength and hope.

### Nursing Diagnosis Statement

#### A. Health Status
Spiritual strength

#### B. Contributing Factors
Appropriate religious education
Firm spiritual identity

Maintenance of belief system during times of
adversity

Maintenance of personal belief system despite
nonacceptance of others

Ability to realistically question religious
teaching

Dynamic belief system

Adaptable belief system

Ability to accept the belief systems of others

Ability to maintain personal values and
principles

Realistic application of religious and moral
principles to a unified philosophy of life

Empathy for other's value systems

Ability to integrate religious teaching into a
personal belief system

Recognition of the need for spiritual assistance when indicated

Deliberating the meaning of life, suffering,
and death

Sense of spiritual fulfilment
Ability to cope with barriers to the practice of
   religious rituals (*e.g.,* hospital restrictions,
   dietary restrictions, and medical procedures)

## C. *Defining Characteristics*
Practices spiritual rituals
Expresses satisfaction with spiritual beliefs

# III
# Case Studies/
# Care Plans

# Case Study/Care Plan 1:
# *Optimum Nutritional Status*

*Case Study:* Mr. Sellers, is a 42-year-old married salesman for an insurance company. He is 6'0", medium frame. Mr. Sellers visits his physican for an annual physical. He is very conscious of incorporating high-level wellness needs into his daily life-style.

| NURSING DIAGNOSIS | GOALS |
| --- | --- |
| Optimal nutritional status (wt = 162 lb) related to availability of adequate resources and wife support in grocery shopping and meal planning/preparation, as evidenced by:<br><br>  Wt = 162 lb— within 10% of ideal body weight for height, build, sex, and age<br>  Absence of fatty deposits<br>  Healthy appearance of skin, hair, teeth, and nails | Over the next year, client will maintain current weight within 5 lbs.<br><br>At next yearly physical, client will report continuation or implementation of healthy exercise regimen.<br><br>At next yearly physical, client will report no gastrointestinal problems or appropriate and effective management of difficulties. |

| NURSING INTERVENTION | EVALUATION |
| --- | --- |
| Examine with client and (wife), current nutritional pattern and preferences. | At 1-year checkup (physical exam) client will: |
|     Encourage continuation of practices by client (and wife) that are supportive of optimal nutritional state | Weigh 162 lb ($\pm$ 5 lb) Report no weight fluctuations or decrease/increase over the past year |
|     Explore practices or preferences with tential detrimental effects on nutritional state | Project healthy appearance (hair, skin, teeth, and nails) Display minimal fatty bulges |
|     Teach client (and wife) about potential harmful effects associated with these preferences or practices | Relate nutrition practices consistent with healthy weight management Relate exercise/activity practices consistent with healthy weight management |

| NURSING DIAGNOSIS | GOALS |
|---|---|

| NURSING INTERVENTION | EVALUATION |
|---|---|
| Assist client and wife to identify healthy alternative choices or patterns | Report no/minimal GI difficulties or effective management of GI problems |
| Collaborate with company or agency dietitian in identifying nutrient content of restaurant selections | |
| Teach client about healthful food selections while traveling | |
| Explore current activity level. | |
| Encourage current level of activity (if appropriate for age, sex, and capability) | |

## NURSING
## DIAGNOSIS                    GOALS

| NURSING INTERVENTION | EVALUATION |
| --- | --- |
| Assess for existing gastrointestinal difficulties. | |
| Teach client (and wife) appropriate intervention measures Refer to appropriate health care provider if indicated | |

# Case Study/Care Plan 2: *Effective Individual Coping*

*Case Study*: Susan Sharp is a well-adjusted, academically talented 8-year-old girl. Susan and her family recently moved to a new area necessitating a change in schools for Susan. She has attended her new school for 1 month with an obvious healthy adjustment. Susan visits the school nurse for her initial school health assessment.

| NURSING DIAGNOSIS | GOALS |
|---|---|
| Effective individual coping associated with successful adaptation to new school, as evidenced by:<br><br>    Development of friendship with two fellow students<br>    Inclusion in play activities during recess<br>    Client states "I really like this school." | During the progression of the school year, client will continue to initiate and maintain friendships with classmates.<br><br>Client will show minimal physical or behavioral evidence of stress during this academic year.<br><br>Client will maintain academic record consistent with ability during the academic year. |

| NURSING INTERVENTION | EVALUATION |
| --- | --- |
| Continue to assess for physical evidence of adaptation to new school (*i.e.*, appetite, elimination pattern, and somatic complaints). | At 3-month interval, client maintains friendships with classmates. At 3-month interval, client demonstrated minimal evidence of stress. |
| Continue to assess for psychological adaptation to new school (*i.e.*, subjective comments, teacher, parent, and classmates input). | At 3-month interval, client demonstrates minimal evidence of stress. At 3-month interval, client shows a good academic record. |
| Collaborate with teacher and parent regarding client's performance and adjustment. | |
| Encourage verbalization of feelings associated with changing schools. | |

| NURSING DIAGNOSIS | GOALS |
|---|---|

| NURSING INTERVENTION | EVALUATION |
| --- | --- |
| Maintain parental and scholastic support of the client. | |
| Provide positive reinforcement to the parents for effective support of client during this adjustment process. | |
| Refer to an appropriate health care provider if appropriate. | |

# Case Study/Care Plan 3:
## Activity Tolerance

*Case Study:* Mrs. Elder is a 78-year-old married woman who lives with her husband and daughter. Mrs. Elder has been diagnosed as having chronic osteoarthritis. She is seen for an annual physical examination at her Health Maintenance Organization.

| NURSING DIAGNOSIS | GOALS |
|---|---|
| Potential for activity tolerance associated with adherence to therapeutic regime, as evidenced by:<br>    Increasing mobility<br>    Understanding of/ and compliance with medication regime<br>    Appropriate rest/activity/exercise program | Over the next 6 months, client's mobility level will increase.<br>At next physical examination, client will report initiation and maintenance of healthy exercise program.<br>At next physical examination, client will report adherence to a medication regime. |

| NURSING INTERVENTION | EVALUATION |
| --- | --- |
| Teach the client the importance of following a realistic activity/rest pattern. | At 6-month checkup client will: |
| | Report an appropriate increased activity level |
| Teach the client a modified exercise regime. | Follow modified exercise regime |
| Teach the client the importance of taking prescribed medications on time. | Take medications appropriately |
| | Express understanding of drug/food interactions |
| Teach the client about drug and food interactions. | |

## Case Study/Care Plan 4:
# *Effective Developmental Progression*

*Case Study:* Tommy, aged 10, has a history of having sustained a severe head injury when thrown from his bicycle last year. Since that time, rehabilitative efforts directed at restoring Tommy's physical and mental capacity to normal have shown consistently positive results. Tommy is being seen in the outpatient clinic for a followup today. He greets the nurse enthusiastically and verbalizes his desire to return to school as soon as possible. Tommy's mother is with him, she sits quietly in the examining room, and offers information only if asked directly by the nurse or Tommy. She does describe the plan the family has developed for Tommy's reintegration into the school system which includes appropriate

solutions to problems such as medication administration during school hours, modification of physical education expectations, and availability of
transportation to late afternoon physical therapy
sessions.

| NURSING DIAGNOSIS | GOALS |
| --- | --- |
| Efficient developmental progression related to the use of rehabilitative resources, as evidenced by:<br><br>    Ability, desire to learn<br>    Opportunities to develop independence | Over the next year, the client will continue to meet appropriate developmental tasks.<br><br>The positive regard and support manifested by the mother will continue for the next year. |
| Potential for successful satisfaction of developmental needs related to supportive parenting | Client will be able to initiate and maintain friendships with peers over the next year. |

| NURSING INTERVENTION | EVALUATION |
| --- | --- |
| Discuss supportive practices by mother/teacher/father and encourage continuation.<br><br>Teach mother various ways to enhance the client's developmental progression, *i.e.*, provision of ability-level appropriate toys, investing in toys with a "maturing value," and so forth | At 1-year physical examination, the client will:<br>    Continue to achieve appropriate developmental tasks<br>    Report satisfying relationships with peers<br>    Evidence continued support of mother, father, and teachers |

| NURSING DIAGNOSIS | GOALS |
| --- | --- |

and problem-solving
ability, as evidenced
by:

> Mother's support
> Successful rehabili-
> tative efforts
> Language ability

| NURSING INTERVENTION | EVALUATION |
|---|---|
| Explore opportunites for the mother to encourage constructive interaction with peers. Offer support and encouragement to parents | |

## Case Study/Care Plan 5:
# Effective Crisis Resolution

*Case Study:* Mrs. K., 45 years old, is seen at the Community Mental Health Center, complaining of "feeling anxious." Mrs. K. is employed as an elementary school teacher. She is appropriately expressive, neatly dressed, and groomed. Mrs. K. relates that her husband lost his job 3 months ago as an executive for a large business firm that was experiencing severe cutbacks. Her mother died 2 months ago and her oldest daughter recently left for college.

Mrs. K. has been functioning effectively at work and at home, however, she "feels edgy and nervous and cries very easily" during the past 2 months. Her

affect is appropriate. Her communication pattern is
unimpaired. Ego functions are intact; appropriate
use of defense mechanisms to assist in coping, ori-
ented to time, place, and person, appropriate reality
contact, memory intact, sensory-perceptual functions unimpaired. Body image is intact, cognitive
processing is intact and functional, realistic insight
into the situation. Mrs. K. demonstrates a moderate
level of anxiety, a positive self-concept, effective
coping patterns, and problem-solving ability. Anxiety level does not interfere with cognition. Mrs. K.

| NURSING DIAGNOSIS | GOALS |
|---|---|
| **Diagnosis No. 1** Potential for effective crisis resolution associated with appropriate coping mechanisms as evidenced by: | Over the next 2 months, Mrs. K will demonstrate appropriate behavior, ideas, and interpretations. |

demonstrates an appropriate attention span and fluency in speech.

Mrs. K's overall physical status is normal as evidenced by: proper eating habits, appropriate height for weight, appropriate rest–activity cycle, although she does complain of some difficulty falling asleep. Mrs. K. demonstrates appropriate fulfillment of her spiritual needs through her chosen religious affiliation and practices. She expressed contentment with spiritual life. She regularly attends church services.

| NURSING INTERVENTION | EVALUATION |
| --- | --- |
| Establish rapport and trust. Convey acceptance and empathy. | At the end of a 2-month period, client will: Express decreased feelings of anxiety |

| NURSING DIAGNOSIS | GOALS |
| --- | --- |
| Effective social functioning<br>Appropriate use of defense mechanisms | Over the next 2 months, Mrs. K. will receive support through a therapeutic relationship. |
| | Within 1 week, husband will be involved in Mrs. K's therapy. |
| | Over the next 2 months, client will identify and utilize effective coping strategies. |
| **Diagnosis No. 2**<br>Spiritual strength associated with an adaptable belief system as evidenced by:<br>    Regular attendance at church services | Over next 2 months, Mrs. K. will continue to receive spiritual support. |
| | Over next 2 months, Mrs. K will continue |

| NURSING INTERVENTION | EVALUATION |
|---|---|
| Use therapeutic communication techniques, *i.e.*, create a safe environment, offer support, and so forth | Report less difficulty in falling asleep |
| Encourage verbalization of feelings. | Experience satisfying communication with husband, peers, daughter |
| Encourage mutual evaluation of progress. | Continue to productively function in social settings |
| Mobilize support systems. | |
| Include husband in therapy sessions. | |
| Discuss use of clergy support to cope with stress. | At the end of a 2-month period, client will: |
| | Express continued spiritual support |
| | Report productive |

| NURSING DIAGNOSIS | GOALS |
|---|---|
| Expressed satisfaction with religious affiliation | practicing religious activities. Over next 2 months, Mrs. K will continue to maintain her spiritual support. |

| NURSING INTERVENTION | EVALUATION |
|---|---|
| | discussions with a trusted member of the clergy |
| | Recognize the support offered by her religious affiliation |

## Case Study/Care Plan 6:
# Effective Family Coping

*Case Study:* Mr. and Mrs. Light visited their Health Maintenance Organization with their baby, Steven, for his 1-month physical examination. The physical examination indicates that Steven is developmentally normal. The assessment indicates that nutrition and elimination patterns are appropriate, reflexes are normal, and Steven has an excellent sleeping–activity pattern.

Mr. and Mrs. Light are adjusting very well to the addition of a new baby to their family structure. Each parent's role is flexible with Mr. Light assuming increased household and child care responsibilities to allow for Mrs. Light's rest needs. Mrs. Light supports her husband in fulfilling his work responsibilities. The parents openly express affection to each other and Steven. Mr. and Mrs. Light report a satisfying sexual relationship with some questions about the best birth control method for them.

| NURSING DIAGNOSIS | GOALS |
|---|---|
| **Diagnosis No. 1**<br>Effective family coping associated with attention to emotional needs of each family member, as evidenced by:<br>  Successful adjustment to meet<br>  Family addition<br>  Flexibility of roles<br>  Spouses' expressed satisfaction with their relationship | Over the next 6 months, the family will continue to adjust appropriately to life-style changes resulting from addition of baby to the family's structure.<br><br>Over the next 6 months, each family member's needs will be adequately met. |

| NURSING INTERVENTION | EVALUATION |
|---|---|
| Encourage the continuation of verbalization of feelings of parents regarding life-style change.<br><br>Provide praise for mutual support and encouragement.<br><br>Delineate the family's method of coping and problem-solving ability. | At the 6-month interval, parents will:<br>  Discuss adaptations made to accommodate life-style changes.<br>  Continue to effectively cope with each family member's needs<br>  Continue to effectively problem-solve<br>  Understand normal |

| NURSING DIAGNOSIS | GOALS |
|---|---|
| | Over the next 6 months, parents will continue to utilize effective problem-solving techniques. |
| | Over the next 6 months, parents will continue to meet the physical, emotional, and developmental needs of a growing infant. |
| **Diagnosis No. 2** Adequate sexual function associated with adaptation to changes associated with chilbearing, as evidenced by: | Over the next 6 months, spouses will successfully adapt to family changes and emerging parental roles. |

| NURSING INTERVENTION | EVALUATION |
|---|---|
| Teach parents normal growth and development of infant and appropriate parenting tasks to enhance development.<br><br>Teach parents health needs and common problems encountered by infants to assist in the recognition and preparedness for minor problems. | growth and development needs of infants<br>Know<br>health needs and recognize<br>minor health problems of infants. |
| Ask family to discuss sexual functioning and identify the areas in which the nurse can provide information. | At 6-month interval, spouses will:<br>    Continue satisfying<br>    sexual relationship |

| NURSING DIAGNOSIS | GOALS |
|---|---|
| Report of satisfying sexual relationship Over the next 6 months, spouses will continue to experience a satisfying sexual relationship. | Over the next 6 months, spouses will continue to manifest expressions of affection and intimacy. Over the next 6 months, spouses will utlize an effective form of contraception, mutually chosen. |

| NURSING INTERVENTION | EVALUATION |
| --- | --- |
| Discuss the energy demands and modifications appropriate in the childrearing period. | Successfully adapt to childrearing demands and schedule |
| Praise family for open expression of affection. | Continue to express affection |
| Provide information on advantages and disadvantages of various birth control measures. | Utilize an appropriate birth control measure |

# Case Study/Care Plan 7:
# *Optimum Physical Fitness*

*Case Study:* Keith is a 15-year-old adolescent who has a history of episodic brochospasm diagnosed as extrinsic asthma in his first year of high school. The school nurse conducts a pre-examination interview with Keith as part of a routine screening procedure for all students requesting to participate in the structured sports activities offered at the high school. Keith tells the nurse that he wants to join the baseball team this year. He had been a member of a community soccer league but had to withdraw because of episodes of wheezing and shortness of breath while playing. He tells the nurse that his mother usually calls the doctor when he can't breath and obtains a prescription for "wheezing" medicine. Keith is very attentive while the nurse performs a respiratory assessment. The findings are normal. He asks many questions about asthma and expresses interest in the nurse's suggestion that they meet dur-

| NURSING DIAGNOSIS | GOALS |
|---|---|
| Potential for achieving optimal physical fitness and activity level associated with adequate respiratory functioning and sense of industry, as evidenced by:<br>    Attentiveness and interest in his diagnosis<br>Effective respiratory functioning associated with clear breath sounds, as evidenced by: | Keith will understand the relationship between sustained activity and brochospasm within 3 weeks.<br>Keith will be able to identify factors that trigger brochospasm and wheezing within 3 weeks.<br>Keith will begin regular participation in self-care. |

ing his study hall period to discuss preventative measures he could utilize to establish better control of his respiratory functioning.

| NURSING INTERVENTION | EVALUATION |
| --- | --- |
| Develop teaching plan for Keith that includes:<br>  Basic mechanism underlying broncho-spasm<br>  Environmental triggers of wheezing<br>  Breathing exercises<br>  Prophylactic use of bronchodilators before exercise<br>Encourage sound health practices<br>Encourage expressions of feelings. | Keith reports a decrease in episodes of wheezing and brochospasm.<br>Keith successfully participates in stop-and-start sports (baseball).<br>Keith maintains a regular exercise schedule<br>Keith maintains peer group socialization.<br>Keith utilizes medication and relaxation techniques as necessary prior to exercise. |

| NURSING DIAGNOSIS | GOALS |
|---|---|
| Findings from the respiratory assess ment | Self-care activities to improve ventilatory capacity within 4 weeks. |
| Potential for independence in self-care associated with high motivational level and supportive environment, as evidenced by: Constructive involvement of mother Willingness to co-operate Inquisitiveness | Keith will exhibit positive adaptation to limitations, self-esteem, and self-concept within 6 weeks. |

| NURSING INTERVENTION | EVALUATION |
| --- | --- |
| Provide positive reinforcement for self-care activities and participation in appropriate activities. | |

# Case Study/Care Plan 8:
# *Effective Elimination Pattern*

*Case Study:* Pamela Elliott, aged 22 months, is brought to the pediatric offices of an urban Health Maintenance Organization. She is accompanied by her mother and is scheduled to have a routine physical examination and developmental screening in preparation for entrance into a day care program. Pamela weighs 24 lbs and is 32 inches tall. Her mother states that she has been walking unassisted for 7 months, has a vocabulary of approximately 30 words, follows simple directions, feeds herself with a spoon, attempts to dress herself, and enjoys imitative play. During the nursing interview, Mrs. Elliott expresses the desire to begin toilet training Pamela, but is unsure of how to approach this task.

| NURSING DIAGNOSIS | GOALS |
|---|---|
| Potential for establishing bowel and bladder control associated with readiness for toilet training as evidenced by:<br><br>    Independent locomotion<br>    Fine motor control<br>    Ability to communicate<br>    Willingness to cooperate and desire to please others. | Pamela will achieve bowel and bladder control within 3 weeks.<br><br>Parents will assist Pamela in achieving mastery of activities associated with control over elimination within 4 weeks.<br><br>Pamela will gain autonomy and positive self-concept through mastery of toileting developmental milestone within 6 weeks. |

| NURSING INTERVENTION | EVALUATION |
|---|---|
| Provide parents with guidance for initiating the toilet training process: | At the next health care visit, Pamela's parents report: |
|    Recognition and observation for Pamela's usual elimination pattern and pre-elimination behaviors |    Daytime bowel and bladder control |
|    Introduction and use of self-toileting practices (*i.e.,* potty chair, handwashing) |    Evidence of Pamela's cooperation and pleasure with the achievement of toilet training |
| Explain Pamela's need for independence and mastery and provide guidance: |    Consistency of approach and reactions to toilet training process |
|    Easily manipulated clothing | |

**NURSING
DIAGNOSIS**                    **GOALS**

| NURSING INTERVENTION | EVALUATION |
| --- | --- |
| Patience | |
| Positive reinforcement for success | |
| Encourage parental consistency and acceptance of accidents or regression during periods of excitement or stress. | |

# Case Study/Care Plan 9:
# *Health Maintenance*

*Case Study:* Kevin, aged 21, was involved in an aggressively enacted football tackle that resulted in the complete fracture of his left femur. Because there was displacement and overriding of the fractured bone ends, Kevin was placed in balanced suspension skeletal traction for 3 weeks prior to surgical repair and casting of his left extremity. Kevin, a well-developed and outgoing college junior, also has juvenile onset diabetes mellitus. He began to assume responsibility for his own health care at the age of 17 after working as a counselor in a summer camp for diabetic children. Prior to that summer, Kevin was frequently hospitalized for episodes of severe hyperglycemia related to noncompliance with his medical treatment program. On admission to the hospital, Kevin was informed about his injury and probable length of stay. While gathering information for care planning, Kevin's primary nurse noted that his main concerns were related to missing his midterm exams and to the interruption of his carefully planned and executed routine of exercise, diet, and insulin therapy. Kevin's family lives in another state and had to return home after his

| NURSING DIAGNOSIS | GOALS |
|---|---|
| Health maintenance: Appropriate related to internal locus of control, as evidenced by: Responsibility for self and autonomous functioning | Kevin will continue to experience a state of wellness during his period of immobilization. Kevin will maintain nutritional status and normal blood glucose levels. |

first 3 days in the hospital. Kevin's roommate, several members of the football team, and his girlfriend frequently visit with him in the evening. Kevin's primary nurse, cognizant of the importance of utilizing patient strengths, included the following positive aspects in what otherwise would have been an accurate but solely problem-oriented care plan for a client such as Kevin.

| NURSING INTERVENTION | EVALUATION |
| --- | --- |
| Provide Kevin with every opportunity for autonomy and independent functioning while in traction. | Kevin considers himself to be optimally well under cirumstances of temporary immobility. |
| Collaborate with Kevin in developing an appropriate and therapeutic routine for his daily | Kevin maintains an uninterrupted sense of responsibility for self and independence. |

| NURSING DIAGNOSIS | GOALS |
|---|---|
| Nutrition status, optimal related to understanding of rationale for dietary modifications (diabetes), as evidenced by:<br>    Diminished episodes of hyperglycemia<br>Potential for optimal nutritional status related to previously appropriate:<br>    Management of nutritionally related problem as evidenced by: Willingness to learn and compliance with restrictions | Kevin will understand and comply with dietary plan designed to prevent complications of immobility. |

| NURSING INTERVENTION | EVALUATION |
| --- | --- |
| living activities while in traction. | Kevin's blood glucose levels are within normal limits. |
| Reinforce knowledge base relevant to dietary modification for diabetic control. | Kevin verbalizes an understanding of the need for increased fiber and protein in his diet. |
| Teach Kevin about nutritional needs associated wtih the prevention of the hazards of immobility. | Kevin makes accurate assessments related to the content of meals provided him. |
| Arrange for consultation with dietitian to assess and plan a diet with Kevin. | Kevin collaborates with the dietitian to plan an appropriate diet. |

| NURSING DIAGNOSIS | GOALS |
| --- | --- |
| Potential for achieving optimal physical fitness related to a sense of industry, as evidenced by:<br><br>    Previous adherence<br>    to a regular exercise<br>    regime | Kevin will understand the importance of activity and exercise while immobilized. |
| Potential for satisfaction of developmental needs related to desire to learn, ability to maintain friendships, and open expression of | Kevin will be able to maintain academic standing and developmental need satisfaction. |

| NURSING INTERVENTION | EVALUATION |
| --- | --- |
| Teach Kevin about the effects of immobility on physical fitness. | Kevin performs prescribed exercises regularly. |
| Educate and plan with Kevin a regular routine of resistive and isometric exercises for unaffected extremities and muscle group. | Kevin does not sustain any of the complications associated with inactivity while immobilized. |
| Arrange for physical therapy consultation as additional support for Kevin's desire to maintain fitness. | |
| Assist Kevin with contacting college professors for remediation or extension to complete work. | Kevin receives assistance to maintain academic standing. |
| Encourage Kevin's friendships by providing him with auton- | Kevin is comfortable and content with visitors. |

| NURSING DIAGNOSIS | GOALS |
| --- | --- |
| feelings, as evidenced by:<br><br>    High motivational level | |
| Potential for effective individual coping related to successful coping with previous stressors, as evidenced by:<br><br>    Ability to express feelings<br>    Adequate support system | Kevin will utilize previous adaptive mechanism to cope with immobility and will validate feelings expressed. |

| NURSING INTERVENTION | EVALUATION |
| --- | --- |
| omy in functioning while immobilized. | |
| Encourage expression of feelings. | Kevin maintains self-esteem and the ability to mobilize internal resources for adaptation. |
| Provide positive reinforcement for previous ability to cope and encourage utilization of healthy adaptive mechanisms | |

# Case Study/Care Plan 10:
# *Positive Body Image*

*Case Study:* Mildred is a 75-year-old, alert, well-educated, single woman who is visited in her comfortable studio apartment in an affluent retirement community. She has recently visited the ophthamologist at the community health center who confirmed her fear that her vision is diminishing. She has decided to have cataract surgery "after the holidays, so I can make the customary family holiday visits first."

In conversation (Mildred is very talkative), it is learned that she cooks one meal each day on her gas stove or oven (the other is eaten in the community dining room) and she is an avid vitamin and health food proponent. She credits her adherence to advice written in *Prevention* magazine for keeping her "pretty well, for an oldster." She states that she also believes in "fresh air, cleanliness, exercise, and R and R" (rest and relaxation). Her apartment is exceptionally neat. She keeps throw rugs at the doorstep "so I don't get dirt in the wood floors after my daily walks" and in the kitchen area "to catch the

| NURSING DIAGNOSIS | GOALS |
|---|---|
| Positive body image associated with appropriate strategies to seek medical treatment as evidenced by: <br>     Visit to ophthalmologist <br>     Appropriately scheduled surgery | Client will have cataracts removed within 2 months. <br> Client will safely cope with diminished vision until scheduled surgery. |

crumbs." She relaxes with a warm bubble bath every evening just prior to bed. She uses the bathroom at least once every night, but is able of returning to sleep without difficulty and sleeps "like a log" for at least 8 hours a night. Mildred confides in the nurse that she is used to being independent and "I hate having people help me because I can't see."

| NURSING INTERVENTION | EVALUATION |
|---|---|
| Support client's decision to schedule surgery at a convenient time. | At the 2 month interval, client will: |
| | Have cataract surgery |
| Teach client safety measures necessitated by decreased visual acitivity. | Safely cope with diminished vision |
| | Explore feelings regarding diminished vision |

# Appendix:
# Data-Base Assessment Guide

This guide will assist the nurse in collecting data to assess the functional health patterns of the client in order to determine actual or potential nursing diagnoses. The following questions can be utilized as a guide in promoting health, preventing illness, and enhancing the strengths of clients and families.

## Data-Base Assessment Format

### 1. Health Perception—Health Management Pattern

- Describe your present health. Is it better or worse than a year ago?
- Do you have any present health concerns?

213

- What positive health practices do you engage in presently? (Your family, your children?)
- Do you smoke cigarettes, a pipe, or a cigar?
- What do you know about the effects of smoking?
- How do you avoid illness and stay healthy?
- What information would you like to have to improve your health (and that of your children, family) and prevent illness?
- Describe any existing barriers to health promotion activities.
- Are you currently taking any medications?
- Do you have any medication allergies?

## 2. Nutrition–Metabolic Pattern

- How is your appetite?
- Describe a typical day's food intake (list any food allergies/food sensitivities)
- How often do you eat at home? In restaurants?

- Describe your food preferences/restrictions.
- Have you had any recent changes in diet?
- Do you take any nutritional supplements?
- Any difficulty in eating/drinking?
- How much fluid do you drink in a day?
- What is your thirst pattern during the day?
- Do you add salt to your food while cooking or at the table?
- Describe your weight pattern over the last 5 years.
- What is your knowledge of the four basic food groups?

## 3. Elimination Pattern

### Bowel

- What is the usual time, frequency, color, consistency, and pattern of bowel movements?
- Do you take laxatives/enemas to have a bowel movement?
- If so, how often? For how long?

- Any recent changes in bowel pattern?
- Any problems with bowel elimination?

### Bladder

- What does your urine look like?
- Are there any difficulties/problems in your usual pattern of urinating?
- Do you experience any burning or foul-smelling urine?
- Any recent changes in urination pattern?

### Skin

- What is the condition of your skin?
- Any problems, irritants, or allergies that you have experienced?

## 4. Activity–Exercise Pattern

- Describe the type and frequency of daily activity.
- What type of job do you do?

- Describe the type and frequency of recreational activities.
- Describe your degree of physical fitness.
- Are you satisfied with your present level of fitness?
- If not, how would you like to change your degree of fitness?

## 5. Sleep-Rest Pattern

- What is your usual sleep pattern?
- Do you feel restored with the amount of sleep you get?
- Any problems or changes in your sleep pattern?
- Do you take naps?
- What do you do when you want to relax?

## 6. Cognitive-Perceptual Pattern

- What activities assist you in resting?
- Do you like school/work?

- If not, describe why.
- How do you usually express your thoughts and feelings to others?
- Do you wear glasses, hearing aid, and so forth?

## 7. Self-Perception Pattern

- Describe yourself. (What do you like/dislike about yourself?)
- Describe your body. (What do you like/dislike about your body?)
- How do you feel about your weight and appearance?
- Have you experienced any physical alterations/changes of your body?
- If so, was or is it difficult for you to accept those changes?
- Have those changes affected your relationship with others?

## 8. Role–Relationship Pattern

- Do you live alone?
- If not, with whom?
- Describe your family (if applicable).
- What are your family's (significant other's) expectations of you?
- What are your expectations of yourself?
- Whom do you confide in?
- Whom do you socialize with other than your family?
- How frequently?
- Are you satisfied with this amount of contact?
- Describe your cultural background.

## 9. Sexuality–Reproductive

- How did you learn about sexual functioning?
- Do you have a sexual relationship with anyone now?
- Are you satisfied with the relationship?

- What birth control measures do you use?
- Do you know how to examine your breasts/ testes?
- What is the frequency of the breast/testicular examination?
- Do you have regular pap smears/testicular examinations?

## 10. Coping–Stress Tolerance

- How do you resolve problems?
- What are the stressors you are presently experiencing?
- Have there been any major changes/losses in your life?
- If so, was or is it difficult for you to accept those changes/losses?
- How have those changes/losses affected your relationships with others?
- What do you do when you are experiencing stress?
- Whom do you turn to for support?

## 11. Value–Belief System

- Is God or religion important to you?
- What is your religious affiliation?
- What are your religious practices?
- What is your involvement with church groups?
- Do you practice the same religion you practiced as a child?
- What is your reaction to people who do not believe in God?

# *Bibliography*

Bircher A: On the development and classification of diagnoses. Nursing Forum, 14:10,1975

Carlson JH, Craft C, McGuire AD: Nursing Diagnosis. Philadelphia, WB Saunders, 1982

Carpenito LJ: Handbook of Nursing Diagnosis. Philadelphia, JB Lippincott, 1984

Gordon M: Nursing diagnosis and the diagnostic process. Am J Nurs, 76 (12):98., 1976

Griffith JW, Christensen P J: Nursing Process Application of Theories, Frameworks and Models. St. Louis, CV Mosby, 1982

Pender, NJ: Health Promotion in Nursing Practice. Norwalk, CT, Appleton–Century–Crofts, 1982

Webster's New Collegiate Dictionary. Springfield, MA, G. & C. Merriam Company, 1974

# *Index*